W9-BAO-435

FORGET THE EXCUSES. JEAN NIDETCH HAS HEARD THEM ALL!

Heredity . . . big bones . . . nerves . . . lack of willpower . . . natural tendency to gain . . . These are but a few common excuses that the overweight use to justify excess pounds.

Jean Nidetch knows them all. In fact, she herself used them when she was a 200-pound-plus housewife for whom all diets mysteriously seemed to fail.

Then she learned how to lose weight and keep it lost, and how to help others do the same. Now she tells just how it can be done—without starvation diets, without seven glasses of water a day, without sunflower seeds, without any of the fads that come and go with every passing year.

And as innumerable women and men who have participated in her program will proudly testify—Jean Nidetch's methods really work!

SIGNET Books of Related Interest

☐ **LET'S EAT RIGHT TO KEEP FIT by Adelle Davis.**
Sensible, practical advice from America's fore-
most nutrition authority as to what vitamins, min-
erals and food balances you require, and the warn-
ing signs of diet deficiencies. (#W4630—$1.50)

☐ **THE ROOTS OF HEALTH by Leon Petulengro.** The
passport to good health is in the natural food that
grows all around in the fields, hedges and gardens. The author tells you how to keep healthy by
using the right foods, truly the "roots of health."
(#T4267—75¢)

☐ **SIX WEEKS MAKE YOURSELF OVER PLAN by
Dolly Wageman.** Here is a unique, easy-to-follow
and fun makeover program that has been developed by leading authorities in the field of exercise
and weight control. (#Q4244—95¢)

☐ **JOGGING, AEROBICS AND DIET: One Is Not
Enough—You Need All Three by Roy Ald, with a
foreword by M. Thomas Woodall, Ph.D.** A person-
alized prescription for health, vitality and general
well-being based on a revolutionary new theory of
exercise. (#Q3703—95¢)

THE NEW AMERICAN LIBRARY, INC.,
P.O. Box 999, Bergenfield, New Jersey 07621

Please send me the SIGNET BOOKS I have checked above.
I am enclosing $_____(check or money order—no
currency or C.O.D.'s). Please include the list price plus 15¢ a
copy to cover handling and mailing costs. (Prices and num-
bers are subject to change without notice.)

Name_____

Address_____

City_____State_____Zip Code_____
Allow at least 3 weeks for delivery

The Story of
WEIGHT WATCHERS®

by JEAN NIDETCH

As told to Joan Rattner Heilman

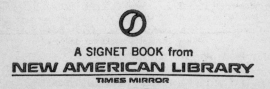

A SIGNET BOOK from
NEW AMERICAN LIBRARY
TIMES MIRROR

Dedicated to my sons, David and Richard:
With love and hope for a bright new world and to
help remind you that you can accomplish whatever
you want to, if you want to badly enough.

COPYRIGHT © 1970 BY W/W TWENTYFIRST CORPORATION

All Rights Reserved. No part of this book may be reproduced
in any form, either wholly or in part, for any use whatsoever,
including radio and television presentation, without the
written permission of the copyright owner. For information
address W/W Twentyfirst Corporation, 635 Madison Avenue,
New York, New York 10022.

Library of Congress Catalog Card Number: 79-111033

"Weight Watchers" is a registered trademark of
Weight Watchers International, Inc., Great Neck, New York.

This is an authorized reprint of a hardcover edition
published by W/W Twentyfirst Corporation and distributed
by The New American Library, Inc., in association with
The World Publishing Company.

 SIGNET TRADEMARK REG. U.S. PAT. OFF. AND FOREIGN COUNTRIES
REGISTERED TRADEMARK—MARCA REGISTRADA
HECHO EN CHICAGO, U.S.A.

SIGNET, SIGNET CLASSICS, SIGNETTE, MENTOR AND PLUME BOOKS
are published by The New American Library, Inc.,
1301 Avenue of the Americas, New York, New York 10019

FIRST PRINTING, MAY, 1972

PRINTED IN THE UNITED STATES OF AMERICA

Foreword

WE LIVE IN AN AGE OF SKEPTICS. There are few heroes anymore. Our kids are anti-hero. They root for everyman and
do battle for the underdog. As we grow older, we tend to
root for virtually no one and do battle for *things* rather than
people. It almost seems that we've forgotten that we have
to have heroes and heroines. So few people seem to come
along whom we can look at in wonder and who can delight
and inspire us.

For most of my adult life as businessman, publisher,
editor and writer, I, like most people, found few who struck
me as being particularly spectacular. Joe DiMaggio could
hit a baseball and John Wayne was strong and bold and
even braver than Errol Flynn. Richard Burton has a fabulous way with women—or, at least, I suspect he has—and
Wilt Chamberlain is as big as the Jolly Green Giant, as
agile as an antelope and as strong as Charles Atlas and
King Kong in tandem. But they're not heroes—they're stars.
Stars are famous and talented and rich and something special. But no—they're not heroes. Not to me.

Billy Graham is a hero to many. He can stand on a stage
and move you to great passion. He can get you to change
your ways and your life. Joan of Arc had to have been a
heroine. Alexander the Great was a hero and so was Lincoln
and, surely, Martin Luther King and Jack and Robert Ken-
nedy and Winston Churchill.

But you don't necessarily have to be known throughout
the world to be a hero and it isn't required that you be a
political or military leader or a religious persuader. Your
own hero could have been your father or your favorite uncle
or maybe the head of Elks Lodge Number 747, the man

who got you to enjoy being with other people. Maybe it was a doctor who gave so much of himself.

Jean Nidetch is not Billy Graham nor, certainly, is she Joan of Arc or Winston Churchill or Martin Luther King. To millions of people who lived all their lives cloaked in a suit of fat, however, she is a heroine.

She has given hope and, more important, fulfillment to people who had given up in despair. She has taken those drowning in their own bodies and shown them what could be done. She has spoken until her voice could only whisper to convince one solitary fat person that he could be like anyone else if he wanted to badly enough and if he tried hard enough.

Her crusade has had no political or revolutionary or religious overtones. It's a pretty basic theme—you can lose weight if you eat properly and if you talk about the problem. She has preached and cajoled and threatened and pleaded and has *convinced* people that they can win.

But don't take her cause lightly. Fat has killed more people than guns. It has killed them physically and killed them emotionally. Jean Nidetch's war is a big one, a bitter one, a serious one. There is at least one overweight person in four out of every five families in the United States. Chew on that statistic for a while. Obesity is a serious contributor to heart disease, high blood pressure, diabetes, and dozens of other major cripplers and killers. It causes mental disorders and, in many cases, virtual withdrawal from everyday society.

Don't write off this war too quickly.

I have seen people weep with joy because Jean Nidetch and the Weight Watchers organization have returned them to the living. I challenge any of you to sit at a Weight Watchers gathering, as I have, and not to react when people walk up to a platform and burst with the pride of being able to say that they have lost 50 or 100 or 200 pounds and that now they can laugh again and play again and walk again.

The book you are about to read is the simple story of a fat woman who discovered how to lose weight and to stay that way and then helped other people do the same thing. Not because she thought she could become rich by doing this—to this day, her mind does not comprehend the intricacies of business or finance—but because she has an enormous enthusiasm for telling secrets and for talking about things and for helping other people who are troubled as she was.

I must confess that I have often been accused of being jaded. It has been said that I'm a doubter.

In 1968, I sat in an auditorium in a Forest Hills, N.Y., high school along with 2,000 other people. Jean Nidetch spoke for more than an hour and then she walked off the podium. As she did, 2,000 people jumped to their feet and cheered and applauded and roared their tribute like the citizens of Rome welcoming Caesar back from the wars.

I suddenly stood very still and was astounded. . . . I had been doing exactly the same thing.

Matty Simmons

Contents

Foreword and Reprise by Matty Simmons

Chapter One

F.F.H. THAT'S ME. Some time ago, I was invited to participate in a seminar on obesity at the Statler Hilton Hotel in New York City. I was the only layman invited. All the others were psychiatrists, psychologists, sociologists, doctors of every kind, and I was the only one who didn't have a bunch of initials like M.D. and Ph.D. to put after my name on the program. So I decided to give myself some. F.F.H. is what I chose: Jean Nidetch, F.F.H. It sounded good.

And that's just what I am. A Formerly Fat Housewife married to a Formerly Fat Bus Driver. I'm also a Formerly Fat Baby, a Formerly Fat Child and a Formerly Fat Girl. I was fat until I was 38 years old, only I didn't call myself fat. I never said the word "fat." I weighed 214 pounds and I was "chubby." But "chubby" isn't for 38-year-olds, it belongs to 18. That's when I discovered I was "big-boned." I carried my "big bones" on a "large frame," and I "carried my weight" rather well. I was a perfect size 44. I surrounded myself with big-boned, large-framed people. I was married to a fat man. I had a fat dog and fat friends. My whole world was fat.

I found out that all big-boned people developed a disease. The disease we had was "glandular." I'm not even sure what "glandular" is, except my doctor said, "You don't have it." But I liked having "glandular" because when a skinny friend would say, "How come you can't lose weight?" I could say, "Glandular," and she would say, "Oh? So, eat something."

It was a great sickness for me, but I made it even worse. I found that "glandular" develops into something more serious called "heredity." My fat was inherited. One of my aunts was very stout—even if she wasn't actually a blood relative.

I used to ask myself, "Why am I fat? I don't eat that much." I never ate breakfast—I got nauseous just thinking of breakfast. I never ate lunch, either. I don't remember ever making lunch for myself. I had two sons and a husband and a house to take care of. I didn't have time for lunch. . . . Well, I did do a *little* bit of eating at noon. You see, when a child goes back to school and leaves some cold French fries covered with cold catsup on his plate, you can't throw them away. If you throw them away, somebody in Europe drops dead. I sincerely hope the people in Europe benefited—I did so much for them.

I had an advantage over most of the fat ladies I knew. My husband, Marty, was fat too. He was 5 feet 10 inches and weighed 265. I was 5 feet 7 inches and weighed 214.

We were *so* jolly. We didn't dance so well together, but we were made for each other as eating partners. We were a hostess' dream. We never complained about the food. As a matter of fact, we got rather excited about whatever was served. Did you ever see a *gorgeous* chicken? Or a *stunning* turkey? A *lovely* cake? *Beautiful* cold cuts?

Somehow, we had a lot of fat friends. It was easier that way because there was always a couple who looked worse than we did. I was always saying to Marty, "Do we look as bad as they do?" And he'd say, "Oh, no, they're sloppy. We're very neat." You know, that's a claim to fame—to be neat!

I was happy except for one thing. There was always one woman at every party who didn't belong there. A size 7. Do you know any size 7's? In my opinion, they have absolutely no personality and, if it's any consolation, I think they age faster than we do. They have no figures and I hate them. But a size 7 was always there. I could always tell because my husband would say, "Why don't *you* get a dress like that?"

I would avoid her, but before the night was over, she would always walk over to me. It was amazing how there could be such a big voice in such a little body. In an unbelievably loud voice, this little thing would say to me, "With a face like yours, how could you let yourself *go* like that?" I never had an answer ready, but I had to say something. I wanted to give her a biting reply. What could I say to hurt *her* a little bit? What could I say to make her go home and envy the way *I* looked? The only thing I could ever think of to say was, "There's more of me to love."

Every night in the bathtub, I would make a promise. I used to promise that I would choke on the next cookie. When you are sitting in a bathtub, there is no place to look. When you look in a mirror, you learn never to look below the shoulders. You concentrate on the face. You tell yourself you have pretty eyes and a nice nose. When you buy clothes, you are very concerned with what's happening at the neckline. When you have your picture taken, there's always a child, a chair, a sweater, *something* to hide behind. But in a bathtub? It's all you and it's floating. You can't escape it. I never took a bath but that I wasn't sure I had been cursed.

Of *course*, I'd been cursed. Surely a skinny size 7 must have come up to my baby carriage soon after I was born and said, "She shall grow up to have a pretty face so that all who meet her will say, 'With a face like yours, how did you ever let yourself go like that?' She shall grow up to be reasonably intelligent, so that the question will hurt. She shall grow up never to eat, but to get fat from *air*. She shall grow up never to take showers but to sit in the bathtub every night surrounded by herself." That was my curse.

After my bath, I'd make the terrible mistake of walking into my living room, where I was forced to look at my couch. Obviously, when you don't like your couch, you have to eat something, maybe a meat loaf sandwich between two slices of salami. Some people think that's ridiculous. For them, it's the carpeting that makes them eat. For others, it's the neighbors. Or the drapes that don't hang right. They'll wake up in the middle of the night, think about the drapes, and they'll eat anything, even if it's stale. Anyway, stale food doesn't count.

After looking at my couch, I would go into the kitchen and eat some chocolate-covered marshmallow cookies.

I weighed 214 pounds in 1961, only I never told anybody. On my driver's license, I always wrote 145. I had never, in my adult life, weighed 145.

That was me, Jean Nidetch, in 1961—214 pounds of big bones on a large frame, suffering from glandular heredity, making promises in the bathtub and breaking them in the kitchen.

In 1962, I lost 72 pounds. And that was the beginning of the Weight Watchers story.

I had dieted all my life. I dieted in preparation for birthday parties. I dieted for graduation. I dieted for my engagement party. I dieted for my wedding. I'm talking about crash diets, any fast method like black coffee with nothing. Or black coffee and cigarettes, or eggs and grapefruit. Oil capsules. Wafers that looked and tasted like dog biscuits. I took little red pills, little yellow pills, little green pills. I lost weight hundreds of times. You can lose weight if you eat watermelon for two weeks. Or bananas and milk, or cottage cheese and peaches. A neighbor tells you about a diet and it works. You lose weight. Sometimes you don't feel well, often you don't look well, but you always lose weight.

I remember one diet where I drank oil and evaporated milk, cold, three times a day, and you mixed it in a plastic container. I don't know why the plastic, unless it was to get the flavor of it. Maybe the idea was that if you suffered enough and if it stuck to the roof of your mouth, you were doing it right. It was called the "Rockefeller" diet. I never discovered why they gave Mr. Rockefeller credit for it, but I remember the recipe. I mixed the oil and milk and drank it all day. It was great. I definitely lost weight. I also got sick to my stomach constantly. My skin had a funny color and my nails got soft, but I lost enough to go off the diet.

After I'd lose 20 or 30 pounds, I'd always go off the diet. That's what a diet is, something to go on and then go off.

But this time, starting in late 1961, it was different. I discovered a new way of eating and a new way of life. I lost 72 pounds—but that's not my claim to fame because I probably could have done that on oil and evaporated milk. The important thing is that it happened eight years ago and I've maintained that loss for eight years. I fluctuate two pounds this side or that, but I never get panicky because I know I'll never be fat again.

I discovered a diet I was told was written by Dr. Norman Jolliffe many years ago. Desperation (I'll tell you about that later) drove me to the New York City Department of Health Obesity Clinic in October, 1961, and there I was handed a piece of paper with a diet on it. I had seen this diet before. All overweight people save diets, it's part of the disease. I studied it like I had studied every other one. The first thought in my mind was that I would rewrite it, change it to suit myself. I would find a way to substitute cake for something else. I'd eliminate the bread and substitute a muffin twice a week. I looked for a way to work in my favorite cookies. I was still firmly convinced that breakfast would make me nauseous.

But I wasn't allowed to substitute anything. I wasn't allowed to cut out anything. I had to go along with the entire program or I wouldn't be permitted to stay with the clinic. And I *had* to stay with the clinic because I was desperate. I had finally come to the point of attending an obesity clinic run by the New York City Department of Health and I was making one last effort to dig myself out of all that fat. I was 38 years old. I had been fat all my life and I wanted to get down to a size 20.

I did get down to a size 20, then a size 18, 16, 14 and, finally, 12. From a perfect 44 I went to an imperfect 12, and I've stayed that way for eight years. I now weigh 142, even less than what it used to say on my driver's license.

I lost all that weight on the obesity clinic's diet, but I added something. I added talk. I found that I couldn't do it on a diet alone. I had to be able to *talk* about my eating problems, to tell other people what I was going through. So I called up a few fat friends and asked them to come to my house to talk. They came. And then they came every week after that, bringing other fat people with them. It was our little group where we met to tell each other about being fat. Soon the group grew—40, 50, 60, 100 people— until now hundreds of thousands of people gather each week in classes run by formerly fat people like myself to talk about losing weight. There have been close to two million members of Weight Watchers so far.

My little private club has become an industry. I never intended it to. It was really just a group, a group for me and my fat friends. But today, there are more than 8,000 Weight Watchers classes held every week in the United States, Canada and many other countries throughout the world. It's as if, never having had a lesson, I sat down at a piano and played a concerto. It's utterly fantastic.

Weight Watchers is now a public corporation. We are in the food business, we have a summer camp for overweight girls and a dozen other projects in the wind. I wrote a cookbook in 1966, called, of course, *The Weight Watchers Cook Book*. It is, I am told, one of the few cookbooks ever to hit the best-seller lists. *Weight Watchers Magazine* has a paid circulation of more than 600,000 a month. It is sold in supermarkets and on newsstands all over the country.

When I am asked how successful Weight Watchers is, I never know how to answer. Do you measure the success of something like this by the amount of money that has been made or by the number of people who have come to you? Are these true signs of success? I think the best way to measure our kind of success is to speak to a person who has lost over 200 pounds. When he tells you how his life has changed, how he's now joined the human race, how he now has self-respect and the respect of his family, his friends, neighbors and the mailman, then you know how successful we are.

I think of the paraplegic who has become one of the best basketball players on his wheelchair team. He used to be so heavy that he could hardly move himself in that chair. . . . I think of the nun who lost 123 pounds and told me that she can now continue to work for God without fear of dying in the attempt. . . . I think of the 8-year-old girl who sent me a valentine that said: "I love you because you helped me look beautiful—I lost 18 pounds."

And the 72-year-old woman in Connecticut who lost 60 pounds and told me: "I feel as if I'm starting my life all over again. Now I'm going to help other people do it." She's on the staff of Weight Watchers International today.

And George, who got stuck in the turnstile entering the World's Fair and had to be cut loose by the fire department. He lost 254 pounds.

The most important thing about Weight Watchers is that hundreds of thousands of people have lost weight with it and have learned how to keep it off. We used to lose weight all the time—and then gain it right back. We were like Yo-Yo's. *Now* we look in a mirror when we've reached our goal weight and say, "This is me and I'm never going to change. I'll never get fat again. I don't have to suffer, I don't have to starve, I don't have to be on a diet. I'm in control of myself."

Now we've learned that we have power over ourselves. Weight Watchers has changed attitudes. We've made a dent in the thinking of the world. Today you can go into a restaurant, the smallest diner or the plushest restaurant and say, "I'm a member of Weight Watchers and I want my fish broiled dry, without butter." You'll get it and with no remarks from the waiter.

You can go to a friend's house for dinner and say, "I'm sorry, I can't eat the dessert. Weight Watchers, you know," and the friend will understand.

When I first started Weight Watchers, I used to think it was all a dream. I thought that all the people listening to me must be doing something I didn't recommend. They must be taking diet pills or injections. They couldn't be losing weight just because I was talking to them, convincing them not to eat layer cake and chocolate cookies.

Then, not too long after, I realized that they *really* were doing it my way. They had become fat the same way I had become fat and they were getting thin the same way I got thin. We were all part of a tremendous army.

When we first started, people would go to a class, and the next day, someone who knew they had been there the previous day would approach them and say: "So? What did you do there? You sang songs? You were hypnotized? What could they teach you that you don't know already? Furthermore, you don't even look any thinner."

Weight Watchers does not simply give you a method of losing weight. What it is, is a new way of life.

Chapter Two

I'VE HEARD PEOPLE DESCRIBE Weight Watchers as "group therapy." I have heard people say, "It must be brainwashing." It's been called "self-hypnosis," a "revival meeting" and "the fat man's Alcoholics Anonymous." I've even heard a woman tell a friend, "I don't care what it's called. I get a fix every Tuesday night." I find I constantly refer to Weight Watchers as a "thing." I simply cannot find the proper words to describe it. It has brought gratification to so many people and yet I have no name for it.

One of our lecturers once said, "It's a place where you walk in fat and hope nobody notices you, and four or five months later, you walk out thin and hope that everyone sees you."

And, other than saying, "It's a new way of life," I've never been able to explain exactly what Weight Watchers is. Basically, of course, there is a diet which must be followed. But I prefer to call it a program, because it is not something you just forget about when you have lost your weight. It's a plan for eating that will stay with you the rest of your life, if you want to remain thin. You will probably eat more than you ever have before, but you will learn to eat in an intelligent, disciplined way, three meals a day with all the "legal" snacks you want between meals.

But Weight Watchers is more than a food program. It's a fat club, the first one that's ever been successful. Actually, what's been added to Dr. Jolliffe's diet is *talk*, it's really not much more than talk. It's people gathering together to talk about their eating habits. When they eat. Why they eat. How they eat. And to be told, by the leader or lecturer of the group, how to eat properly.

It works. Compulsive eating is an emotional problem

18

and we use an emotional approach to its solution. To me, this is just plain common sense.

The biggest reason Weight Watchers is such a success is that fat people can finally talk freely, openly and honestly. We can reveal our real feelings to other people and those other people will understand. I can say to a Weight Watchers class, "I remember sitting in a bathtub watching my fat floating," and there isn't a person there who can't relate to me at that moment. A thin person would never understand that.

I once heard a woman say to a friend during a class, "Mabel, we can take our coats off here." Now, this was a great thing to her. *Here,* in *this* place, she could take her coat off without embarrassment. Obviously, there were other places where she and Mabel never removed their coats. Obviously, they were ashamed to show what they looked like. *Here,* they could remove the lie, the façade they had been living with for so long.

Before Weight Watchers, fat people couldn't communicate with thin people and they couldn't communicate very well with each other, either. Fat people were the biggest bores in the world. No one cared what they did or didn't eat for lunch. No one cared whether they had two hors d'oeuvres or 25 hors d'oeuvres at a party. A thin person couldn't understand. If I were talking to a brunette, would I dare talk about what I go through to make my hair blond? She wouldn't have any interest in the fact that every three weeks I devote a whole day out of my life—plus money, effort and some discomfort—to it. How could she possibly understand and why would she care? If I told it to another blonde-by-choice, she would be interested and might even have some helpful advice.

Empathy, rapport, a mutual understanding are the keys. Fat people didn't always tell the truth, even to each other. But now they do. They have a reason to. They learn to be honest and open with each other because *somebody else* starts first. . . . It began with me. I told my friends that I ate cookies in the bathroom at night. The first few times, you could hear the gasps. They were shocked that I could admit such a thing.

The honesty is like giving away a whole, total recipe. Did you ever know women who never tell another woman a complete recipe for anything? They always leave out one ingredient, so you can't make it come out right. Not me.

If I knew of a store that was selling two quarts of milk for the price of one, I told everybody. If I found out how to make a delicious orange cake, I spread the news. And if I weren't the kind of person who gave what I found to others, I would never have told anybody what I'd found at the Department of Health, and there would never have been Weight Watchers.

All you need is one person in a group to be honest, and then, slowly, very slowly, everyone else starts telling the truth. That's why our lecturers must be former members of Weight Watchers, they must have lost weight *our* way. Then they can stand up there in front of a class and tell the group about themselves, about their own eating problems, their own success in losing weight, their own ability to survive without eating promiscuously. That starts the ball rolling and encourages other people in that room to stand up and talk. It's such a relief to be able to talk about something we never really discussed honestly before, about the anger we feel, the secret longings we have, the private eating habits we indulge in. Here we talk to other food addicts. Who else can you tell that you eat cookies in the bathroom at night? Who else can you tell that your mother used to make sure that you ate everything on your plate? ("Clean your plate, there are starving children in Europe." I bought *that* line for a long time.) Who else can you tell that your husband (or your wife) doesn't find you appealing anymore and that you are desperate to win him (or her) back?

We can finally *say* the word "fat." We don't have to stand up at a meeting and say, "I am fat," but we must know that that's what we are and we must say it to ourselves—"fat," not "chubby" or "pleasingly plump." We're really saying it when we walk through the door of an organization dedicated to overweight people. It takes courage to open a door that says Weight Watchers on it, or anything else that means "this is for fat people." We're telling the world that we are fat and we are desperate. We've exhausted every other known method there is. We're not beginners. We're professional dieters.

Once people start talking honestly, they always discover that somebody else in the room does exactly what they've been ashamed of doing all these years. They find out they aren't the only ones who eat peanut-butter sandwiches on the way to the supermarket, or sneak downstairs in the middle of the night to gobble up a loaf of bread and a dish of macaroni salad by the light of the refrigerator.

"My God!" a woman once said at a meeting, "I ate a cold lamb-chop sandwich last night!"

One woman spoke up in a class a few years ago and said that one night the week before, she'd gone to Nathan's (a famous stand-up eating place in New York) all by herself and waited at the window for service. The man inside said, "How many?"

She didn't know why, but she said, "Four." So he gave her four hamburgers, four hot dogs, four bags of French fries. She ate everything.

When she told this story in a Weight Watchers class, nobody laughed, nobody was shocked. Everybody felt compassion for her. They all knew they might have done the same thing.

When my children were young, we used to hire a baby-sitter occasionally. The baby-sitter was a skinny little girl from across the street. I remember buying strawberry shortcake for her one night and saying to her as I left the house, "There's cake in the refrigerator for you and some ice cream, too."

I'm going to admit something now that I never admitted before Weight Watchers existed. When we returned that night, my husband took the sitter home. While he was gone, I went to the refrigerator and took out the strawberry shortcake. The sitter hadn't eaten it—she was a skinny little size 5 or 7 and she'll never be fat in her life because, as a rule, she'd never go within three rooms of strawberry shortcake. In the few minutes Marty was out of the house, I picked up the cake in my hands and devoured it.

And I'll tell you what was worse. When Marty got back, I said to him, "How do you like that? She ate a whole cake while we were gone." So, in one moment I became a thief and a liar. I was lying to my husband, who was fat, too, and really didn't care what I ate. But I couldn't even admit it to an ally. And I wanted to say something nasty about that skinny kid because she could sit in a house where there was strawberry shortcake in the refrigerator and ignore it. She could live without it. To me, eating strawberry shortcake was a real emotional experience.

I used to tell that story at our early classes and it would

always open up a hornet's nest. Everybody would start telling stories about the terrible things they had done.

In a group like this, you can brag too. You can tell the others in the class that you went to a dinner party and you *didn't* eat the hors d'oeuvres. Where else can you be acclaimed for such a marvelous deed? Where else can you brag about passing up a piece of chocolate layer cake? Here you can do it and everyone is happy for you.

Chapter Three

I DON'T KNOW IF I will ever discover exactly what obesity is, but I know what it isn't. It isn't funny. It isn't a sin. It isn't ignorance. It isn't stupidity. Being fat has nothing to do with being dumb or smart. I knew *why* I was fat and what to do about it, but I needed something to make me do it.

Being fat isn't a disgrace. It isn't big bones and a large frame. It's rarely a glandular problem or heredity. It isn't stout, chubby, pleasingly plump. It's fat, *fat*, FAT.

Currently, statistics reveal that one out of every five Americans is overweight and about 20 million people are dieting at any one time. And statistics tell us that obesity is one of the major killers in our country. The fat man who constantly stuffs himself is literally killing himself. He could drop dead from a heart attack or a stroke, but even worse, he could die emotionally. I've met fat people who were emotionally dead. I've met people who looked as if life were all over. They've given up. They're ashamed and afraid.

There are teen-agers who have never roller-skated or gone bowling or ridden a bicycle or gone out on a date. There are children who hate to go to school because their classmates tease them mercilessly. There are men who don't drive a car because they can't fit behind the wheel. There are boys who want to enter a profession but can't get into college because of their excessive weight.

You never see some fat people. They never go outside. They stay home because they can't walk without getting out of breath and they can't climb on a bus. You never see them at the movies because the seats are too small. They don't even go shopping because people laugh. They order their groceries by phone or send someone out for them.

There's a wonderful girl in New Jersey who has lost 125 pounds so far on the Weight Watchers program. When I met her, which was just recently, she weighed 600 pounds. For 12 years she had been a recluse, never leaving her home. One day, she was listening to the radio and heard me talking. That very week, she went to a Weight Watchers class, just walked in and sat down and felt at home at last. Now she is on her way to success and I've promised to be there when she graduates at her goal weight of 155. She'll make it.

Most people, of course, don't have such an enormous problem. Some only need to lose 25 pounds, others, 50 or 60, but all of them worry about going to the beach or getting up on a dance floor where everyone can watch and make the classic comment: "My, isn't he light on his feet?"

Fat people aren't the jolly types you might think they are. They've got a problem and they know it. They're not jolly at all. They're angry. That is, they're angry by the time they come to us. They're angry because everyone else gets what *they* want: the jobs, the dates, the compliments.

My husband and I developed a beautiful comic routine —we were very funny in public. But I wasn't funny when I sat in the bathtub and looked at myself. I wasn't funny when I caught a glimpse of myself in a store window. Marty was the funniest man at any party, but he never took off his robe at a swimming pool until he got to the very edge of the pool. The robe was dropped there and the minute he got out of the water, he put it right back on. That took a lot of thinking. He had to plan ahead.

When you're fat, you are constantly plotting and planning. For example, you always eat something before you leave your house. This is so that other people never see you eating too much. I was never brave enough to sit there, all of me, big and fat, and eat myself into oblivion if I knew there was one skinny person in the room staring at me.

The first thing I'd say to my husband when I'd walk into a roomful of people was, "Am I as fat as she is?" pointing to some other big woman. And he would say, "Of course not. And even if you are, you're taller. So, you carry it better."

Fat people are not fancy eaters. We get used to picking

up whipped-cream cake with our hands because we don't want to leave dirty forks as evidence. We are not delicate eaters—we eat with a passion. Watch fat people in a restaurant—it's as if the whole meaning of life is there on that plate in front of them.

Fat people are always urged to eat; somebody is always offering us more food. Hostesses who have spent the day preparing a gourmet meal insist that tonight we go off our diet. Our parents urge us one day to lose weight and the next day say, "I worked so hard on dinner. Eat the pudding!" A waiter comes over, who couldn't care less, and says to the fat man, "We have coconut cream pie today." He doesn't say that to the skinny fellow, because he's not so sure he'll want it, but the fat man is sure to order it. Even if he has told himself, "I'm going on a diet today," he wants to please the waiter and his diet can wait a little longer, so he orders the coconut cream pie.

Fat people think they can't do anything right. A fat salesman is sure he's not going to make the sale if there's another fellow bucking for it. A real-estate salesman said to me, "Not only did I lose 60 pounds, but now I sell more houses. I know I didn't learn anything new about real estate since then, but my business has picked up. It's got to be because nobody takes you seriously if you're fat, especially yourself."

A fat person is always treated like some kind of freak. He's talked to differently. He's looked at differently. It's hard for anyone else to understand, but everything he does is different. One man told me, "Nobody really listens to what you say when you're so fat: You look stupid. Everyone expects you to trip over things: You look clumsy. Everyone expects you to spill your soup: You look sloppy."

There are other problems. When you're fat, there's the fear of spring, when you know the warm weather is coming and you won't be able to cover yourself up with a big coat any longer. There's the humiliation of going to a party and knowing that you look worse than anybody else, though you may be younger and prettier and smarter. There's that uncomfortable feeling that your clothes are squeezing your insides together.

There's the fear of the comments you hear from well-meaning people. I used to cringe when someone said, "If you'd just lose some weight, you'd look great."

There's the knowledge that every so often you'll catch

a look on someone else's face just at the moment he first sees you. You're afraid of the amazement, perhaps the revulsion you'll see there.

I remember the carousel. Do you know that as a child I never got up on a horse at the carousel? I used to sit in one of those stationary wagons with the grandmothers. I would say I didn't like the horses, but I did. I was just afraid people would laugh at me.

When I went shopping for clothes, I didn't look for style, I looked for anything that would go around me and that had something interesting going on at the neckline.

I remember, whenever I was offered a lift home, I was always concerned about how many people were going to be in the car. Three in the back seat? I might not fit.

Today, fat people still worry about fitting into the car, they still worry about finding clothes that will go around them. But they have discovered that so many other people have the same problems. You'd be amazed how it helps, just to know that.

Chapter Four

I'M JUST A FORMERLY FAT HOUSEWIFE. I'm not a doctor or a psychiatrist. I'm not a dietitian. I don't know any of the technical details of nutrition, and I never had lessons in hypnosis, nor have I been to an A.A. meeting.

But I *do* know how to eat, how to lose weight and stay that way.

I don't guarantee that losing weight makes life beautiful. I don't guarantee that it's going to give you the success in life that you want. But *surely* it's going to make you confident that you are capable of controlling your own body, that you are not the victim of your compulsions.

Except for the relatively few who do have medical problems, most people who say they don't know why they are fat aren't telling the truth. They *do* know. And you must admit it, at least to yourself, because it's such a relief to be able to say, "I'm fat because I eat too much." In most cases, there's no mystery about being fat. It comes from overeating the wrong foods.

Fat people are always potentially fat people, even when they're thin. We aren't like "civilians," those people who are thin without trying. We have a problem—*we must keep eating*. When civilians have a bad day, their throats lock up and they can't eat. When they're angry, they can't eat. When they're in love, they can't eat. It's just the opposite with us. We're *compulsive eaters* and we *must* keep stuffing food into our mouths. We'll probably never be any different. The answer is that we have to learn to stuff the *right* foods into our mouths.

Not too long ago, I learned the word "appestat." The appestat is like the thermostat in your house. It's set at a level at which you feel comfortable. When you've eaten enough, your appestat should turn off your appetite. When you eat less than your appestat is set at, you feel hungry. When you eat more, you feel full.

Normal people have appestats that work properly, but the obese individual's appestat is faulty. It doesn't shut off when he's eaten enough. I used to be able to eat endlessly. There seemed to be no bottom; I was never satisfied.

I don't know if you know what halvah is. It's a kind of creamy, crumbly candy. I'd take a slab of halvah, put it between two pieces of bread and make a sandwich—a halvah sandwich. It was a marvelous concoction. Right now, it makes me drool to think about it. I remember dozens of times, after eating a huge meal that had come after a whole day of nibbling, when I'd go into the kitchen and make myself a halvah sandwich.

Compulsive eaters have to learn that food isn't the answer to all our problems. It's fuel, that's what food is; it's a necessity because without it we can't function. But pleasure and rewards must come from other sources.

Compulsive eaters always say, "I can't lose weight." Until Weight Watchers, I said it. Everybody in the world accepted it when one of us said, "I take after my mother." Or, "I eat like a bird. It's my metabolism." Sure, we eat like birds. A bird eats four times its own size. Better we ate like horses. Quite frankly, I don't know what metabolism *is,* but I know that mine is normal.

You *can* lose weight, but you must decide if you really *want* to. If you're fat and it doesn't make you unhappy, go ahead and stay fat. But stop talking about losing weight. Stop saying, "I don't know what it is that makes me so fat. I wish I could lose weight." Stop traveling around to doctors for new pills. Forget it. Adjust to it. Accept it and learn to live with it. You are going to be the way nature made you—fat.

But if you're fat and it's destroying you and you really want to lose weight, how much are you willing to give to do it? Money? Not enough. Ten miles of traveling each way to reach a class? Not enough. Can you give up a peanut cluster, or a gumdrop, or a piece of pizza covered with anchovies and sausage? *That* will do it.

Compulsive eaters *can* lose weight—and it's very simple. Look, it doesn't matter how smart you are. Even a Phi Beta Kappa is capable of selecting a chocolate cupcake instead of a stalk of celery. He may be a student of nutrition and know that celery is better and safer, but he'll still choose the cupcake. Why? Desire. We can't diminish that desire. It's there and it's very real.

But we can help him *replace* his desire for cupcakes with a desire to get thin. In that same person, there's a desire to wear pants without pleats, to play basketball, to go dancing and not feel ashamed of how he looks. A desire for cupcakes can be replaced by a desire to look good. In other words, vanity.

There is no more compelling reason to lose weight. Occasionally, a person comes to our classes because his doctor says he has to have surgery but must first lose 100 pounds. Occasionally, someone joins because his blood pressure is so high that he is in danger of having a stroke. But even if it is for a serious, medical reason, I've discovered he really comes because he wants to look better. Vanity is the reason 99 per cent of the time. I never could get all choked up about the health benefits of proper eating habits. I never cared about nutrition. But I did care about how I looked.

I have always felt that if someone were to tell me that smoking would cause a disfiguring mark on my face, or a rash to break out all over my body, I probably would have quit smoking long before I did. Fear of cancer wasn't enough. It's the same with obesity. People have been told they were going to die because they were fat, and it hasn't been enough to motivate them to lose weight. But let someone say, "You look ugly," and maybe then something will happen.

If strawberry shortcake made you break out in purple spots, you wouldn't eat it. You'd be allergic to it. But, do you think fat is prettier than purple spots? It's uglier and harder to get rid of. You *are* allergic to strawberry shortcake and pizza and chocolate. They make you break out, not in purple spots, but in fat.

If you can keep in mind, when you are tempted to eat chocolate cookies in the car going to your mother-in-law's, that you hated to look at yourself in the mirror that morning, you can solve your problem. If you can keep in mind, when you are handed a rich dessert or a serving of French fried potatoes, that tonight will end and tomorrow morning will come and you will feel heartbroken because you can't wear the clothes you like, or because you can't look at yourself in a mirror without wincing, you can solve your problem.

Everybody talks about willpower. What is it? It's something I used to say I didn't have. Most people hide behind their lack of it. They'll say, "I haven't got willpower," and that ends it. This gives them the right to be fat or alcoholic or anything else.

I tell people who walk through our doors, "It was willpower that brought you here. So, obviously, you have this thing you thought you didn't have. If you've got the courage to join Weight Watchers, certainly you've got the courage to put back a cupcake, certainly you've got the courage to let go of a doughnut, by all means you can pass up a pretzel."

I think "desire" is a better word than willpower. I have the desire now to be thin and it's greater than the desire to eat the sweet foods I love. I have the desire to wear a size-12 dress and it's greater than the desire to stuff myself with chocolate-covered marshmallow cookies.

You can be surrounded by French pastry and you can love it. You can look at it and want it . . . but you can't *eat* it unless you pay the price. And the price you pay is fat.

You know something? Your own birthday cake is not fattening. You can hold it close to you, you can smell it, you can serve it. It's not fattening. It's only fattening when it gets into your stomach. It gets into your stomach via the weapon that's attached to your wrist. You're in control of the weapon, so blow out the candles, serve the cake to your guests and then have half a grapefruit. Your stomach doesn't know it's your birthday.

At a meeting one night, a woman said, "I gained weight last week because I entertained, and I've simply got to taste everything I serve." I told her that a wine taster is not intoxicated all the time. The wine goes only as far as his taste buds and doesn't go down his throat. I said, "If you want to taste the food you're making for your guests, where is it written that you must swallow?"

I don't believe you lose your love for cake just because you give it up. I still yearn for rich desserts. I still look longingly at hot-fudge sundaes. I still drool when I watch a TV commercial about a cake that's extra-moist and delicious and easy-to-make in your own kitchen, and it's being sliced right there in full color in front of me. I still salivate when I leaf through a magazine and see a picture of chocolate cream-filled cookies; or when the doorbell rings and a neighbor says, "Here, taste this. I just baked it."

But I want a size 12 more than a piece of cake. I look at cake and I see a size 44. I look at a cantaloupe and I see size 12.

One 10-year-old girl wrote me not long ago that she had a weakness for bread and what should she do about it? I told her that an extra piece of bread gives pleasure for only a few seconds, but being thin is enjoyable all the time.

Obesity is a war and we who are fighting it daily are well aware of the turmoil and strain of battle. You win the battles by developing a tremendous desire for something that's more important than cake—being thin.

If you feel strongly about having a body that you like, then surely you don't have to love cottage cheese, surely you don't have to get excited about a tossed salad with lemon juice, surely you don't have to lose your cool over a strip of green pepper. You simply have to love the end result, to get excited about the finished product. I never thought I could enjoy a cup of coffee without a Danish. They went together like a frankfurter and a roll. But I've learned to eat the frank without the roll and to enjoy the coffee without the Danish because I love the end result.

Fat people say to me, "I'll never make it." They'll make it if they take it one step, one battle, one crisis at a time. Don't give up the whole thing if you can't make it the first time. Just like when you were learning to walk, you'd fall down a lot. If you hadn't gotten up and tried some more, you would never have accomplished the tremendous feat of walking. It's the same with losing weight. Just remember that other people have had the same problems and have done the same thing. Just start again.

Is it worth it? Well, I go to the beach and I'm not embarrassed in a bathing suit. I always was before. I go shopping and buy whatever clothes I like. I never could before. I enjoy tennis and I'm learning to play golf. Would I have been seen on a tennis court or a golf course before?

I used to eat my rewards. Now, the reward is self-respect. It's worth it.

Chapter Five

I WASN'T ALWAYS FAT. The day I was born in Brooklyn, on October 12, 1923, I weighed 7 pounds, 3 ounces. A nice medium-sized baby. But I started getting fat the very next day. It was stylish in those days to be a fat baby. It was cute. And it was particularly cute to be a roly-poly little girl. I didn't mind it a bit.

I'm sure that my compulsive eating habits began when I was a baby. I don't really remember, but I'm positive that whenever I cried, my mother gave me something to eat. I'm sure that whenever I had a fight with the little girl next door, or it was raining and I couldn't go out, or I wasn't invited to a birthday party, my mother gave me a piece of candy to make me feel better. And she must have said, "Stay home and I'll make chocolate pudding," for somehow I learned that food would fix any hurt. And that it would celebrate any joy. I know that's what must have happened because it's what I did with my own children.

My father was always thin and my mother was heavy. We all used to joke with my father because he didn't eat and he was so thin. He just didn't care about food. The doctor gave him an appetite stimulant, but he always forgot to take it. He was a cabdriver and he usually didn't get home in time to eat dinner with us. But my mother would wait up for him and serve him dinner at 10 or 11 o'clock, and eat with him, again, to get him interested in his food. She would always ask him, "What did you have for lunch today?" And he'd usually say he'd forgotten to eat lunch. That used to strike my sister and me as very funny. How could anybody *possibly* forget lunch?

Food was always very important to my mother, my sister and me. Lamb stew was my favorite. You could have a fabulous time with lamb stew, there was so much to it. On Sunday, which was a big day because my dad was home, we always had steak and French fries. Thursday was vegetable-plate night. It always included corn and potatoes, and chocolate pudding and cake for dessert. I ate all the other stuff to get the desserts. For years, whenever I served anything to my own family that wasn't meat, I always made at least two desserts.

Daddy was the strong one in our family and we all leaned on him. We respected him and we loved him. He was very funny and there was always a lot of laughter when he was around. He had a limp and had to wear high, clumsy shoes, but somehow when I think about him I rarely remember that. I knew he was perfect.

He was always dreaming about doing something big. He was enterprising, but he never really made it. One year, during the Depression, when the WPA workers were all over Brooklyn, he came up with the idea of selling sandwiches to the work gangs. Mother made the sandwiches and he piled great stacks of them in the back of his car along with a tremendous urn of coffee and a load of paper cups. In the mornings, before he drove his cab, he sold the sandwiches and coffee and managed to make extra money.

We lived not too far from Eastern Parkway, a very wide street. One summer, Daddy thought, wouldn't it be something if he could sell ice cream to the people who sat on the benches along the parkway every afternoon? Instead of having to get up and walk to the candy store, they could buy their ice cream right where they sat. So, he bought an old beat-up truck and painted it white. On the panel of the truck he wrote "Wonder Bar" in red letters, and he hung a bell over the windshield. Then he went to an ice cream plant and bought pops and cups and put them in a freezer in the back of the truck. My sister, Helen, and I would print stars on every 10th pop stick and the child who got a star would trade the stick in for a little football or a doll. Daddy made enough money to pay off the truck that summer.

But then the weather turned cold. People didn't want ice cream on the street when it was cold, so Daddy went back to the cab again. The next summer he planned to return to the ice cream business, but this time he'd buy a couple of bicycles and hire boys to sell in other areas for him while he covered Eastern Parkway.

My mother was a sweet, hard-working woman who was completely dependent on my father and left all decisions to him. She was a manicurist and worked several days a week in a local beauty parlor. Sometimes, when I was small, she'd hire a girl to take care of my sister and me while she was at the beauty parlor. The girl was usually a farm girl from somewhere upstate and wouldn't stay very long.

Since we were living in three rooms then, Helen and I slept on a pull-out bed and the girl had a roll-up cot, all in the living room. My parents had the bedroom.

Sometimes, now, when I feel a little guilty about being a working mother, I remember that my mother worked, too, and I'm sure it didn't hurt us at all. In fact, I think we loved her even more because when she was home, it was wonderful.

Today, somebody's always asking me, "Now that you're a career woman, when do you spend time with your children?"

I answer, "Would you believe that I think I spend more time with my children than when I was a housewife?" When you're home all the time, you're always looking to get out—so you join clubs or a card group, or you take courses. If you manage to spend time with your children, it's haphazard and you usually don't pay too much attention because you're busy cooking dinner. Now, my time is planned. When I know I'm going to be out of town, I deliberately make plans to be with my boys the weekend before. And I'm home most nights for dinner.

I think every working mother feels guilty sometimes, but often she finds the children don't care as much as she does. Our David, for example, has reached the age where it's, "Hi," or, "Good night, I'm going out." And that's that.

My sister, Helen, who is four years younger than I, was very thin until she was about 4. Then she had her appendix out and started to gain weight. I don't know what an appendectomy could have to do with gaining weight, but she gained. Now there were two fat girls in the house. My mother would introduce the two of us like this: "This is Jean, who was always chubby. This is Helen, who was never chubby until her operation." We were both fat, but Helen and I were very different and we still are. She was a mischievous little thing and I was a worrier. She had olive skin and dark hair. I was fair.

As I got older, I was still a "lovely, chubby girl." I don't think I was too troubled by it, because you know how families pamper the fat kid—they pinch her cheeks and feed her candy and cookies. The thin child gets a stuffed bunny for Easter; the fat one gets a chocolate bunny because people think this is what she wants.

The biggest problem I had was finding clothes that fit. There were certain stores that sold "chubbies" for young girls like me, but the clothes weren't pretty and I never liked them.

I was always on a diet. My mother disapproved of appetite suppressants and so did our doctor, but I went on fad diets. For a whole week, I would eat just one kind of food or nothing at all. I would get angry and irritable and I weighed myself every hour on the hour. I'd lose a little, but then I'd give it up and eat more than ever to make up for my deprivation. Or I would diet by *not* having five ice cream pops every afternoon.

My mother learned how to serve diet foods. She would give us broiled meat, green vegetables and salad. Never potatoes or bread. But then, because we were so good and ate our dinner, we'd usually have a rich dessert. Mother enjoyed eating, and being overweight herself, she couldn't be too strict with us.

In high school, I was still the same way, though I don't remember people saying I was fat. Chubby, yes. Never fat. By the time I was 15, I detested the word "chubby." I was popular because I was a talker and I developed a circle of friends, all overweight. Occasionally, I would truly like a thin girl, but I didn't want to become too friendly with her because she could never understand me. I did have one thin girl friend, Evelyn, who, like me, spent her lunch money on ice cream. Instead of buying milk and a sandwich, we would each eat five ice cream pops for our 25 cents. How she got away with it, I'll never know, but she ate what I ate and never had a weight problem.

I never liked gym class. The fat girl is never chosen for a team, and—oh—those green bloomers! The elastic should have been placed about the thigh, but I pulled mine way down to my knees to cover up my fat legs. I used to play sick so I could skip gym, and I soon decided I wasn't the athletic type.

Dating didn't start until rather late. I was about 16 or 17. Even though I was fat, it wasn't a bad time for me. I usually dated fat boys anyway—they made me feel smaller, I guess.

I wanted desperately to go to college. I didn't know what I wanted to be, but I was determined to be someone important. I received a partial scholarship to Long Island University, but I couldn't accept it because we couldn't afford to pay the rest of the tuition. So I decided to go to City College of New York and take a business administration course.

It was February, 1942, and college had barely begun for me. Daddy had had a cold for about three days and was looking so terrible that my mother finally convinced him to go to the doctor. By the time he got there, he had a collapsed lung. He died in the hospital four days later. He was 42.

It was a terrible shock. I remember, when I went out after the mourning period was over, being so surprised that the trolleys were still running and people were still going about their business. Why hadn't the world stopped?

My mother was 36. She had two young daughters and was very much on her own. Fortunately for her, if there is any good fortune in such a thing, she had a trade. She immediately took a full-time job as a manicurist.

Of course, I had to quit college and go to work. I got a job with the Mullin Furniture Company in Jamaica, N.Y., earning $10 a week. Helen quit school, too, lied about her age and found a job as a cashier in a movie house. I was 18 and Helen was 14. We all became very concerned about each other, and very close. We were frightened and confused because we'd lost the one person we'd all relied on. I became the strength of the family because I had to: Mother turned to me automatically and Helen was really just a kid.

Later I went to work for a company called Man O'War Publishing. It published a tip sheet for horse players.

During those years, New York had a most unusual and exciting mayor, Fiorello LaGuardia. When Mayor LaGuardia was not reading comics on the radio during a newspaper strike or doing other colorful things, he was very busy trying to close down anything related to horse racing. During this crusade, my life was changed. One Saturday morning, two young men arrived at the Man O'War office and, before anyone realized what was happening, they told us the place was ordered closed by the police "for further investigation." I never found out what happened after that because my boss suggested that maybe I should look for another job.

So I began working for the Internal Revenue Service, where I stayed for five years until I got married.

I was living at home in Brooklyn. My mother was re-married in 1946, to a very nice man whom I admired very much. Mother, Irving, Helen and I lived together until April, 1947, when I got married and left for Oklahoma.

I don't know how it is at the Internal Revenue today, but when I worked there, there was lots of free time. There were coffee breaks all day long, so I ate all day long. And I can remember coming home from work on the subway and stopping in at the delicatessen downstairs from our apartment before I went up for dinner. I was too hungry to get up the stairs without a hot dog on a roll or a piece of pastry.

While I was working there—it was 1945—I met Marty. I was 21 and he was 27. He lived in my neighborhood and I met him in a luncheonette where the owners knew us both. When we were introduced, I was having a Danish pastry with coffee. Marty had been out of the Army for a month and he had the distinction of being one of the few soldiers who had liked Army food. He told me he ate everything and loved it. If some of the other soldiers didn't like what they got, Marty would eat it. He always carried a couple of onions in the pocket of his uniform to cut up into the rations to improve the flavor. He was fat and he worked at being fat.

We ate together. We didn't go dancing or bowling or roller-skating. We ate. We traveled long distances to special restaurants and thought nothing of waiting half an hour for a table. We weren't gourmets. So long as it was plentiful and filling and tasty, we loved it.

Up to that point, I was fat, but I wasn't too bad. I fluctuated between a size 18 and 20. Until very recently, I told everybody who would listen that I wore size 18 when I was married. That was a big thing because I was a 20 when we became engaged. I struggled with black coffee and cigarettes to make the 18, but I have to admit now that it had to be let out at the sides.

Marty and I went together for two years. When we decided to get married, I went to my grandmother's house to tell her. She was happy. She said, "Of course, I knew you would marry him. He's just right for you."

I adored my grandmother. She was sweet and gentle. For years and years, I visited her every Friday night. She was hard of hearing and she didn't wear a hearing aid, so I had to shout at her. The neighbors used to think there was a fight going on.

Grandma was an understanding old lady. I never talked to anyone the way I used to talk to her. She always gave me encouragement. I found a friend in her and we'd sit and talk for hours, the two of us shouting back and forth at each other. I think she was really my most intimate confidante. I'd go to her house right from work on Fridays. It became a ritual.

I loved listening to Grandma's stories about how she met and loved my grandfather. He was the only man she ever loved in her life. They lived in a little town in Russia where things were very bad, so after they married (she waited seven years for him until he got out of the army) and had five children, Grandpa came to America. When he'd saved enough money, he sent for her and the children. Two of them, twins, died on the boat coming over. My mother was the oldest of the children, about two or three months old when she came to America. Another baby was born in this country.

Grandpa was tall, very distinguished looking and powerful; Grandma was tiny and frail. He sold pickles and herring and sauerkraut from a pushcart in the Wallabout Market in Williamsburg in Brooklyn. Later he rented a corner store and sold pickles in barrels. They were poor, but they worked hard and were terribly devoted to each other.

Grandpa was very religious. Grandma was religious, too, although she didn't go to services often. She said you don't have to go to a temple to be religious, you can be religious in your own home. To her, religion was being good to other people, giving of yourself.

Grandpa died in his 50's when I was quite young, and his tiny little wife lived many years longer. I used to tell Grandma all about my love life. I'd tell her I'd met a boy and she'd ask, "Do you like him?" And I'd say, "Oh yes, I do. I'm sure I'm in love." And she'd say, "He's for you. I know he's for you."

And the next time, I'd tell her I no longer liked that

boy, that we'd broken up. And she'd say, "I knew he wasn't for you. He wasn't your type. You'll find the right one for you." For Grandma, whatever I wanted was right.

I miss her. I miss those talks we used to have. She died in her sleep about 10 years ago when she was well into her 80's. She had moved to Lakewood, N.J., to live with my mother's sister.

After I got Grandma's approval of our marriage, we started to make plans. Marty was working as a blouse salesman in New York, but he got an opportunity to be credit manager in a store in Tulsa, Okla. It seemed to us like the perfect way to start a new life.

Marty went to Tulsa to see if he liked the job and to find a place for us to live. While he was gone—it was a couple of weeks—my mother, sister and I planned the wedding and sent out invitations.

When Marty returned, everything was prepared. It was a simple affair and we invited about 50 people. The wedding was at 5 in the afternoon, in a little temple that was right next door to my grandmother's house. There was just a buffet table, but it was a nice wedding. I wore a navy blue dress (the size 18 with the sides let out). Fortunately, in 1947 the bustle was in style and it covered plenty in the back. The dress was long, almost to the ankles, because that was the style then, too—the New Look.

I really went overboard on the hat. When you're fat, you go overboard on hats and shoes. I always had difficulty finding shoes. My feet were so big that there wasn't very much else I could do except buy anything that fit. But that hat! I went to a shop in Brooklyn on Utica Avenue and paid $30 for it—and this was in 1947. That's like $100 today and I'm sure it was more than the dress cost. It was a big beige cartwheel and I still have it. Holding on to mementos is one of my traits. If anyone ever wants to see the first picture taken at Weight Watchers, or our first newspaper article (or the 3,000th), or a telegram I received on a birthday, I've got it. I'd like to frame everything that holds a place in my heart, but since the walls are never big enough, I simply save it all in boxes and albums. Looking through them relaxes me now almost as much as eating used to.

Seeing that big cartwheel, my mother said, "What are you ever going to do with a hat like that in Tulsa, Oklahoma, with the cowboys and Indians?"

Tulsa, Okla., to a Brooklyn girl who had never been away from home even for a weekend, was the other end of the world. The only thing I knew about Tulsa was from a movie that had cowboys and Indians, and oil wells gushing all over the place. In that movie, only the cowboys wore hats.

A friend at the Internal Revenue Service, where I had been working until the wedding, was a woman who was related to Barbara Stanwyck. She said to me, "For luck, I'm going to get you a pair of Barbara's gloves to wear at the wedding." In 1947, Barbara Stanwyck was the biggest movie star in Hollywood and she was married to Robert Taylor, who was my idol. I knew those gloves had to be lucky.

Chapter Six

THE WEDDING WAS on April 20, 1947. The next day, we left for Tulsa and I felt just like a pioneer. Everything was strange and new and wonderful. We drove west in a 1942 Buick convertible, stopping at every carnival and fair along the way to cram ourselves with hot dogs, cotton candy and soft drinks, and send postcards to our mothers.

It took us a week to get to Tulsa. Marty had rented a furnished room for us, a pleasant room in a lovely house on Quincy Street, owned by a middle-aged couple, Lydia and Owen Seed. The Seeds had no children and were delighted to have honeymooners stay at their house. They were so hospitable to us that I felt right at home even though we were over 1,000 miles from Brooklyn.

We could use the kitchen at any time, but in those days I wasn't much of a cook. You don't have to be much of a cook when you're fat, you know. You can put salami and cheese, and whatever else you can get your hands on, in a roll and enjoy it with a cold drink. It's always easier to have a piece of packaged cake than it is to cook something. You can buy cake anywhere, and pretzels and potato chips are available at every little store, so I didn't do much cooking in Lydia's kitchen.

Our first morning in the Seeds' home, I decided I was going to make breakfast for Marty. I made a fried egg, toast and coffee. Marty walked into the kitchen with a big smile on his face, sat down at the table and then looked at the egg. He stared at the egg. He said, "Look what you've done."

I bent down and looked at the egg.

He just sat staring at it. I begged him, "What did I do?"

Suddenly, he jumped to his feet and walked out of the house.

I was completely distraught. *I* sat there staring at that egg for a half hour, then I got up and called Marty's mother in New York. I told her what had happened.

"Did you break the yolk?" she asked. I told her I had.

"That's it," she answered solemnly.

She told me that when Marty and his brother were young, she had tried all sorts of games to get them to eat. There were tricks and rules. One rule was that the yolk of a fried egg must never be broken until you eat it. Otherwise, it would be bad luck.

To this day, Marty insists on a perfect fried egg, and when he gets one with an unblemished yolk round and clear as the sun, the first thing he does is stick a piece of toast in it!

One reason we weren't in Lydia Seed's kitchen very much—aside from my lack of cooking ability and the fact that fat people can eat right out of packages—was that Owen's favorite dish was boiled eels. Lydia boiled them in a big pot with onions and they were on the menu a couple of times a week. When the eels were cooking, the odor kept us a good distance from the kitchen.

Marty was credit manager for the Federal Store in Tulsa. It wasn't really his kind of job—he's too soft-hearted. But the store was part of a chain and the idea was to prepare Marty to be a manager someday.

Everything was going pleasantly, but I had nothing to do all day. I didn't know anyone except the Seeds. So I got on a bus one afternoon and I went to Main Street and into the first department store I saw. It was called Street's. (By the way, not only did they wear hats in Tulsa, but they wore gloves in the afternoon, too.) I said to the personnel manager, "I'm a saleslady. Do you need any help?" I had never been a saleslady in my life, but I just had to get a job. It wasn't that we needed the money so badly—we were managing because we didn't do very much besides eat and go to a movie once in a while. Of course, we didn't save any money either, because neither of us knew how. I wanted a job because I was bored.

The personnel manager hired me and I worked on a small salary with a commission. The first week I was there, I doubled my take-home money with my commission. I sold a lot of clothes because I invariably made friends with the ladies who came in. I never forced a sale. I always felt that it was better to make a friend than a sale. So, if I didn't like what the customer was trying on, I'd tell her it didn't look good on her. I'd take her phone number and I'd say, "When something comes in, I'll call you." And I did. As a result, I developed a steady clientele. They waited for my phone calls and usually they bought what I recommended.

We'd been in Tulsa for not quite a year when, in January, 1948, Marty was offered a job as manager of his own store in Warren, Pa. By this time, I was rather homesick and the thought of Pennsylvania delighted me because it was closer to Brooklyn. Not only that, but the summer of 1947 in Oklahoma had been the hottest they'd had in 25 years. For more than two weeks there was no rain and the temperature never went below about 116. I didn't look forward to another one of those, although I'd come to love Tulsa.

Shortly before we left Oklahoma, we had moved out of our furnished room into a little furnished house. It was my first house, so I took pictures on the porch with a pot, with a mop, and then with a broom. I baked my first cake there and I have a picture of that, too. When I think back, I realize the house was really almost a shack. But we loved it despite the fact that the girl who owned it came over every Sunday to make sure we didn't move her furniture around.

And, of course, we were fat. You have to remember that. We found great pleasure in ice cream cones. We found an ice cream parlor and we'd go there every night after dinner. And in Tulsa they had watermelon stands. The watermelon was brought to your car on a big tray, tremendous chunks of it, deliciously cold.

When Marty was offered the job in Warren, we decided immediately we would accept. On his birthday, January 20th, we got in the car with all our belongings and left. As we traveled north, it began to get very cold. Marty reached down to put on the heater, turned the knob and nothing happened. We stopped and he looked under the dashboard to check the heater. There wasn't any. (We'd never had to use the heater before because we'd never needed it in Tulsa.) That car was a convertible and without a heater we nearly froze. It was below zero most of the time. But we wrapped ourselves in all the coats we owned and just kept driving, with no stops, to Pennsylvania.

We arrived in Warren one night about 10 o'clock, just

about frostbitten, with the wind whistling through the thin top of the car. We were in a city where we didn't know a soul, and we had everything we owned in the back of the car. We owned very little, only our clothes and personal possessions, but they took up the whole back seat and the trunk. We checked in at the Carver Hotel, which has since burned down. It was a bitterly cold night—Warren is the Icebox of the North, the coldest part of the state—and it was quite a change from Tulsa. Warren's population was 15,000 and hadn't changed in 50 years. All around the edge of the town were farms. We were told that the New Process Company, a mail-order firm, was the big employer there. It's a beautiful town, nice and small and, well, I guess the word is, homey. We liked it right away.

The next morning, Marty and I went to the Federal Store and met the traveling man from the New York office. Marty was introduced to the two salesladies and that was it. The place was his. The store sold everything— refrigerators, furniture, vacuum cleaners, shoes, hats, men's clothes, women's clothes, children's clothes, stockings, you name it. A general store. Everything but food and everything on credit. It looked like Macy's to us because it was Marty's store.

I decided to work there, too—for nothing, to help Marty out and also to keep busy and to meet people. We joined a lot of local organizations—the American Legion, for instance—for the same reason. The store was quite large, but we were only really busy on Friday nights. Otherwise, people just trickled in and trickled out.

Friday nights were the best. That's the big night in a credit store in a small town. All the people come in from the surrounding communities to look around and shop. It was fun. After a while, people used to come to the store just to talk and meet their friends and then buy a few things.

The very first day we were there, a couple came into the store and introduced themselves. They lived in a house owned by the girl's father and upstairs from their apartment was another apartment with three rooms. It was an old house that had been converted into smaller units. They offered it to us and invited us to dinner and to services at the local temple on Friday night. We moved right in. There were only about 30 Jewish families in all of Warren and the arrival of another Jewish couple in town was important to them. That's why they came—to help us.

The very first Sunday after we moved into the apartment, there was a knock on the door. Two ladies stood there, one of them holding a tray of cookies. They were the Misses Alexander who lived next door, and the cookies were for us. From that moment, I fell in love with Warren and I still love it. I fell in love with a town that could welcome you with an apartment and a tray of cookies. I felt like I belonged there, that it was home.

Warren has snow from October until April. It's beautiful snow. It's crisp and clean and it's white, but it's also winter and it's cold. In the apartment we had an oil stove with a pipe that went through the ceiling of the living room. That, plus an electric heater in the bedroom and one in the bathroom, was the heating arrangement.

One night soon after we got to Warren, we went across the street to a small restaurant for a cup of coffee and a Danish after we closed the store. The man who worked in the restaurant (today, he and his wife own two restaurants in Warren) was Bill Proukou. He sat down with us and asked us where we were living and how we liked the town.

As he talked and told us about his wife, who'd just had a new baby, he decided maybe we'd like to meet her. "Come on home with me now. I'm sure she's waiting up for me." So we went to their house. Irene put the coffeepot on and we sat there until 3 in the morning, the baby's feeding time.

Bill and Irene became our closest friends in Warren. There wasn't a night that we didn't see them. They were Greek and through them we not only met more people, but we learned about the Greek traditions and celebrated all the Greek holidays.

Our overweight was taken for granted. Nobody seemed to mind it. I don't think I minded it in those days because we were happy, jolly people. We ate a lot. Irene drank coffee constantly and didn't need to eat. But she made *psomi,* the Greek bread, and *baklava,* that Greek cake with nuts and honey. I flipped over all this stuff. What we didn't finish on our nightly visits, we took home. With Irene a great baker and Bill a good cook (because of his restaurant background), life was one big eating binge.

Marty and I kept getting fatter and fatter. We just relaxed and ate whatever we felt like eating, which was plenty. I blamed it first on marriage. Well, that's ridiculous, you know that. But you have to be able to give a reason for being fat. I blamed it on happiness. The truth was, I just ate. I ate anything and everything. And then, of course, as the children came, I blamed each successive 10 or 20 pounds on them.

We lived a very social life in Warren. There was not much to do or many places to go, so we had to invent things. For no reason at all, somebody would have a formal dinner party. Or a bridge luncheon. Or a tea, or a picnic. Or a George Washington's birthday party. I remember inviting everybody at the temple to come to our house after services on a holiday. Everybody came to our three rooms, 30 couples. They sat on the floor and I opened whatever was in the house—crackers and cheese and cookies and fruit—and everybody had a ball.

Eating, in this kind of place, became a very important part of our life. In a small town, there are usually one or two department stores and that's it. There's only one movie house and you've always seen the picture. You can't go shopping all day. You have a luncheon and you hit the two stores and you go home. So, eating at home with friends was the big pastime.

We learned a good lesson in Warren. Sometime in the first couple of weeks at the store, a man called up and asked, "Do you carry men's hats in a size 5⅞?" It was the smallest size you could possibly get for a man.

Marty said, "No, we don't have that size."

The next day, a woman called and asked, "Do you carry size 5⅞ in men's hats?" And, again, Marty said no.

A couple of days later, a boy came in and asked for that same hat size. I said to Marty, "You know, I don't know this town, but obviously most of the men here have small heads. I think you'd better order that size from New York. Everybody seems to want it."

He said, "Well, let's wait and see. That's a very strange size." Within a couple of weeks, we got about 15 more requests for the same size hat, so Marty sent a wire to the New York office: "Send two dozen size-5⅞ men's hats. Tremendous need here in Warren." The hats arrived and we put a huge sign in the window: "We now have size-5⅞ men's hats."

And we waited. The next Friday night, a family walked into the store—a man, his wife, his children, a grandfather, a grandmother, the whole family. The grandfather, an elderly gentleman with an obviously small head, bought one hat and they all left. They bought one hat, and 23 hats in size 5⅞ were still there when we left the store five years later. Obviously, we had just met everyone who had been calling to ask about 5⅞ hats.

It taught me a lesson. When Weight Watchers started and a woman would call me and say, "You really should have a Weight Watchers class in this neighborhood in the Bronx. We need you." I would say, "Okay, we'll open there as soon as we can."

Then, maybe a few more women would call, but I never forgot the hats. I'd say to Marty, "There's always a possibility the whole family is calling for this one poor soul who needs help." So we waited until we were sure.

But we did get stuck once, anyway. A member of our staff said to me one day, "We've got to open a classroom in this area in Brooklyn. The demand has been fantastic."

I asked if she had a list of names and addresses of the people who were interested. "It could be the old hat story. It could be that everybody's calling for one person."

She said, "But a day doesn't go by that we don't get a request to open in that area." So, we decided to do it.

Two people showed up.

Since then, before we open a class, we make sure of the need. Opening in an area is not simple. You have to rent a room or a hall, buy furniture, take out insurance. You have to send a staff there and do some advertising. Today when we train people to open locations, I tell them the hat story and advise them not to get carried away by a barrage of requests.

I continued to work in the store until I got a job at Sylvania Electric. I was in the personnel department and took charge of the payroll. But on Friday nights I always went to the Federal Store.

There was sadness for us in Warren, too. It was there we lost a child. He's buried in a cemetery just outside of town, called Babyland. It was my first baby and he lived only 36 hours.

I had wanted a child very badly. Everybody we knew had children. It took me two years to become pregnant— possibly because I was overweight—and we were so happy when it happened. And my mother was thrilled and my in-laws were thrilled and Grandma was thrilled. This was to be her first great-grandchild. And the first grandchild for both our families and the first niece or nephew (my sister was unmarried at the time, and so was Marty's brother).

It was a normal pregnancy with no special problems. I went to a doctor who was the only obstetrician in Warren and a good one. He was young and brand-new in town. I was in my ninth month when I woke up one night feeling sick. I went into the hospital and vomited for 14 days. Nobody knew what was wrong with me and they couldn't stop the vomiting. It got so that the movement of the baby would almost throw me out of the bed. I was being fed intravenously, but I was becoming sicker and sicker. The doctor decided he had to induce labor because I was dehydrated to the point of complete exhaustion.

The baby was born and he seemed perfect and strong. He was born crying. And I stopped vomiting. Marty called New York and my mother and mother-in-law soon left for Warren to be with us. Marty and Irene Proukou were with me that entire night and everybody was very happy. I was very weak but starting to feel better.

They didn't bring the baby to me because, as the nurse explained, he was weakened by my vomiting and had to have oxygen. But he was fine.

Marty was sitting by the bed. Suddenly, I felt as if someone had hit me on the head with a hammer. It was a sensation I can hardly describe, but I can feel it now—it was a tremendous jolt. I grabbed my head. And that's when the doctor came in the room. He was visibly upset.

I said, "Something happened to the baby." He couldn't speak. I knew then the baby had died. He just simply expired, they told me later. Then, something strange happened. I saw Marty and I saw the doctor. I saw everything, and I saw them talking. But I couldn't hear them, I'd lost my hearing.

There had to be a birth certificate and a death certificate, and a burial. Marty and Irene took care of all that.

I remained in shock and couldn't hear for some time, even after I got back home. After a few weeks, when I finally could hear again, my mother and I decided to go to Florida to recuperate. But it was December, the height of the Florida season, and we lived in Warren, Pa., and had very little money.

We found an ad in the local paper that said, "Anyone

wishing to share expenses driving to Florida, please call."
We called and discovered that the man who had placed
the ad was a minister in Warren, a fine gentleman who was
going to Florida to visit his daughter. He was driving and
he wanted someone to go along and share expenses. We decided to go.

But we neglected to do two things. We failed to find out
what kind of driver the minister was and we forgot to ask
where in Florida he was going. The only Florida we knew
was Miami and it didn't occur to us that there was any-
place else. We got in the car with the minister that day
in December and left. We were excited because it was a
"first" for both of us.

That man was unbelievably cautious. He drove as slowly
as possible. There were times we went 25 miles an hour—
and it took us five and a half days to get to Florida. He
also didn't drive at night; at 6 o'clock he always stopped
at a motel. So, for five nights Mother and I had to pay
motel expenses, plus our food and our share of the gas
and oil.

The minister was a very pleasant man, quite charming
and elderly. At one point he said, "Oh, darn!" and then he
turned around and said, "I beg your pardon, ladies. I don't
usually swear." He was a fine man, but he cost us a lot of
money. When we had almost depleted every penny we
had, we found ourselves in St. Petersburg on the western
coast of Florida.

"Well," he said, "this is where my daughter lives. Good-
bye and good luck."

We said, "St. Petersburg? Where's St. Petersburg?"

We arrived in St. Petersburg at 6 in the evening and
asked at the bus station how to get to Miami. There was
a bus the next morning at 7, and eight hours later we
would be in Miami. So we checked into a hotel, then
got on the bus the next morning and traveled for eight
hours through the Everglades to Miami.

When we got there, we were in Miami, not Miami
Beach. We wandered around looking for the beach, but
the whole place looked like Manhattan. Nobody told us
that you had to take a bus over to the beach. It was late
by then and we were exhausted.

We were afraid to check into one of the hotels because
they all looked like the Waldorf to us and we were almost
broke. We stopped a woman, simply stopped a woman

who was walking along the street, and my mother said, "Can you help us? We need a place to stay." I don't know whether we looked sad or what, but she said, "Come with me." She took us to the rooming house where she lived in Miami and we stayed there that night.

The next morning, of course, we discovered Miami Beach and Collins Avenue, and found a rooming house on 12th Street. It didn't cost very much. Marty converted his G.I. life insurance and wired me the money, about $500.

It was on this $500 that we stayed in Miami Beach for about five weeks. We had a hot plate in our room and we cooked there. There was a public beach and we had the sunshine, and we had Collins Avenue to wander around on. Mostly we just sat in the sun and wrote letters home.

One day, I met a girl on the beach who had lost a child, too, and we talked about it. Talking was a great consolation. I had never known anybody who had had this experience before and I felt nobody in the world had such a hurt. It's a peculiar kind of hurt, one that you can never forget. It makes you sad and it makes you angry. My mother used to console me by saying, "If you had taken that baby home, if you had learned to love it, to touch it and care for it and *then* lost it, it would have been worse." I would reluctantly agree that it could have been worse.

After five weeks, we went home by bus, tanned, fatter and feeling much better. My mother went home to Brooklyn, I went to Warren, and we all resumed our regular lives.

Then in 1951, I became pregnant again, and I went back to the same doctor. The pregnancy was a tremendous strain on all of us. The minute my mother knew I was pregnant, she came to Warren and spent seven of the nine months with me.

David's delivery was a trying time. When they wheeled me into the labor room, I began to relive the first experience, and when I was wheeled into my room after the delivery, I opened my eyes and saw I was going into Room No. 7, the same room I had been in before. I was convinced the baby had died. But the doctor came to me immediately and showed me the baby and said, "Jean, we have a robust, healthy baby." He was a beautiful baby and he thrived.

Warren was our home and we loved living there, but that was where I got so terribly overweight. All those dinner parties and late-night visits with the coffee and cake were hardly good for my shape. On top of that, David was a poor sleeper and woke up frequently during the night. Of course, every time I got up with him, I'd have something to eat. I'd eat while I was waiting for the bottle to warm, I'd eat while I was rocking him in my arms. When his sleeping habits improved, my eating habits didn't. So, even after he decided to sleep well, I still found myself getting up in the middle of the night to eat.

When David was two months old, we decided we missed New York and we would take our chances on a new life there. Although I was sad to leave Warren, I didn't realize until years later that this was perhaps the best decision we could have made.

Chapter Seven

THE THREE OF US—Marty, David and I—returned to New York in the middle of February, 1952. Marty looked for a job, but it was difficult to find anything. We moved in with my in-laws. When the landlord complained about so many people living in that apartment, we moved in with my mother. Then we moved back again. My mother-in-law had four rooms, my mother had three. And the three of us made it pretty crowded in either place. The general idea was to move quickly and often so as to confuse the landlords.

While we were still at my mother's, I went into the egg business. My aunt used to have a chicken farm in Lakewood, N.J. She'd send me eggs and I'd sell them to neighbors. I started out with a few dozen a week, and then a case. Before I was through, I was getting three cases of eggs a week. I discovered that if you candle them yourself, you can buy them cheaper than if they are already candled. So I bought a candler. A candler sounds intricate, but there's really nothing to it. It's just an unshaded light bulb that sits on a stand with a little indentation in front of the bulb where you place the egg. If you look at an egg with the light behind it, you can see if it's clear inside. If an egg had a spot in it, my customers didn't like it and so I sold those to the bakery where they didn't mind. Doubtful eggs I put in a box and sold to my family and friends. If they got an egg they didn't like, I would replace it.

I started my egg business by going to apartment houses in Brooklyn and knocking on doors. I told the people that I sold eggs, that I would come every week and bring them fresh eggs from New Jersey. All I needed was one woman in a building to say yes, and I would go next door and say, "I'm the egg lady. Mrs. Greenberg next door buys eggs from me. Aren't you interested, too?" I built up a big clientele this way and I sold eggs for about a year. During the day, Marty was job hunting and I was home with the baby. At night when he was home, I went out with the eggs.

I sold in a predominantly Jewish neighborhood and when the Passover holidays came, women ordered six dozen, 12 dozen, 14 dozen eggs. It takes 12 eggs to make a sponge cake for Passover. How was I going to deliver all those eggs? I just couldn't handle it. I was tired of lugging egg boxes around even though they hid my figure— fat girls will carry anything they can hide behind. So I asked Marty if he would be interested in taking over the business. At that time, he was being considered by Carey Limousine Service for a job as a bus driver and he wasn't at all interested in selling eggs door-to-door.

I didn't know what to do. Finally, I went to the post office and bought as many postcards as I had customers and I spent the whole next day writing: "Your egg lady is out of business. Happy Passover." I closed up my little account book and put the candler away. Do you know anyone else who has put herself out of business because things were going too well?

Marty started working for Carey and stayed for 12 years. He drove the limousine buses, the big airport cars that take people from New York to the airports. He was happy there. He was a careful, safe driver and won the safe driving awards year in and year out. He was happy and funny and everybody loved him.

Meantime, we both grew fatter. I tried to lose weight— constantly. I became a professional dieter. Each time I got an invitation to go anywhere, whether it was a wedding or a family circle meeting, I went on a diet. I think there are as many diets as there are fat people. I'd lose 30 pounds and then, the night of the function, I'd say to myself: "Now I've finished the diet and I'll never gain weight again. My stomach must have shrunk." And I'd relax and start eating. You know, you go to the buffet table and help yourself and if the waiter happens to pass behind you, you find yourself reaching with one hand for the buffet and with the other hand for his tray. You do it for fear of starving to death, I guess, and "to please the hostess," who couldn't care less.

So, you're off the diet. That's the horrible thing about diets. And when you go off a diet, if you are born to be fat, as I obviously was and am, you've got to keep going back on one. It's like making a blonde out of a brunette. You have to keep going back for touch-ups.

I exhausted every possible method of losing weight. Eggs and grapefruit, cottage cheese and peaches, bananas, etc., etc. A neighbor always gave me a new diet. Watermelon and black coffee was another. That's a beauty, because you're full all the time. Eat enough watermelon and you're really filled up. And you lose weight. You also get sick after a while.

Then I went through the polly seed phase—this routine came from somebody who *knew*. She said if you eat polly seeds you lose weight—and you do. You really lose weight and you're very busy all day long opening all those seeds, and it keeps you occupied and you're not thinking about anything.

I remember traveling from Brooklyn to New Jersey to a physician who was highly recommended by my neighbor. He gave me an injection, the contents of which he kept secret. It was $10 a visit and it took hours to get there and hours to come home. He said, "Eat anything you like. I guarantee you will lose weight." I lost 45 pounds, but one day I fainted in the street. When I was brought to a doctor, I was completely dehydrated and he said, "You've got to build yourself up. Drink whole milk." Wonderful! I had permission to eat again. So I gained 55 pounds.

For a short period, I went to a hypnotist. I only went for two visits because I couldn't really bring myself to cooperate. It seemed rather ridiculous. He said, "If you place your hands on your stomach, you'll get the feeling you are full." For me, it never worked.

I dieted, lost, gained—and never got down to where I could wear anything less than an 18 dress. The epitome of success was a size 18. That was rock bottom for me. I took appetite suppressants until I was grinding my teeth so hard at night that I'd wake up with a toothache in the morning. I tried anything anybody suggested.

When I wasn't on a diet, we were happy. For years, Marty never brought me perfume for a present. He brought me candy. It was nice, because I loved candy. If we had an argument, if it was my birthday, or Mother's Day, whatever, I never got a sexy nightgown, I never got jewelry or flowers. I got peanut clusters. He'd never give me peanut clusters now, but then I was delighted. Marty knew the secret to my heart. He ate the clusters, too, and we got fat together.

It was "fun." We were "jolly." We developed a whole act about our size and we were the life of every party. People waited for us to say something funny, and we usually did. After all, if you're fat, you have to make a joke about your weight before somebody else does. You have to show that you recognize you're fat and you don't mind it. If *you* say it, it's a joke. Your opening line has to be something like: "I just went off a diet that didn't work." Or, when the polly seed diet was popular, I'd say, "Do I look like a Polly? I've gone on a diet of polly seeds. You can see how it works."

Recently, in an elevator in an office building, I was among seven passengers. Someone remarked that the elevator seemed crowded although the sign said "Maximum 10 persons." A very overweight man commented, "You must understand, I'm really three people." I felt so sorry for him, and I am willing to bet that when he got to his floor, his desire to eat something was overwhelming.

Marty's favorite line, as he patted his stomach, was: "I got this when meat was cheap." It got a laugh. Soon, somebody would say, "Come on, let's eat. Do you think this cake will go with your diet? If not, we'll write a new diet. It'll be all cookies and candy and cake and nuts." Looking back on it, it was sad and not always funny. But people would laugh.

I've seen thousands of "before" pictures of fat people and, it's amazing, but most of the people are doing something comical. The "after" pictures, the thin ones, are usually dignified because then they don't have to do anything but look good. They don't have to put lampshades on their heads.

I remember one girl who had lost 110 pounds. In her "before" picture, she wore a muumuu (every fat woman's boon because it just hangs over everything and in the pockets you can always carry some pistachios) and had a towel draped over her face. She was standing with her hands on her hips like the town siren. She told me, "You know, I remember the day that picture was taken. I wanted to cry because I knew how monstrous I looked, so I had to do something silly."

That reminds me of a costume party we went to in Warren. I think it was April Fool's Day. Neither Marty nor I could get costumes that fit, so we made our own. Marty went as a Chinese man. That was simple—he wore the top of his pajamas over his trousers, a coolie hat, a long cigarette holder and a big black moustache. I don't know if a Chinese man ever looked like that, but we thought Marty was fine.

I went as Bloody Mary from *South Pacific*. I took the drapes off the living room windows and wrapped them around me. Then I got a big straw hat and added the wax fruit from the kitchen table. I was Bloody Mary and she was fat, too, and it was great. We were unbelievable, but we told stories about fat Bloody Mary and her Chinese fat man and everybody laughed.

We moved to Deepdale Gardens, an inexpensive co-operative garden-apartment project, in Little Neck on Long Island in 1953. Now we were living in "the suburbs," surrounded by grass and trees.

In 1956, I became pregnant again. By this time, I weighed 190 pounds. My obstetrician said, "If you don't lose weight during this pregnancy, I guarantee you a heart murmur when you're through."

I tried to lose weight, but of course I couldn't go on any of my crazy diets when I was pregnant and I couldn't manage to stick to any sensible way of eating. As a last resort, the doctor recommended appetite suppressants and, although I probably was malnourished by the time Richard was born, I weighed 30 pounds less than before I became pregnant.

We were a fine family and I was at my thinnest in many years. The old eating habits returned, however, and before long I was fat again. Of course, I taught the children how to eat and David was a good student. He was a healthy baby and he was a fat baby. When he was an infant, the "experts" didn't believe in pacifiers. So, if you can't give a child a pacifier, what better thing can you give him than a piece of bread or a pretzel?

I didn't eat breakfast—I don't remember ever eating breakfast. As a result, David was always a poor breakfast-eater. I knew children should have a good breakfast, so I encouraged him to eat one. But children are great imitators. He didn't like it and often went to school without any at all.

David would eat everything else, though, just as I taught him. I used to say to him, if he had a fight with another child, "Don't feel bad. Have a lollipop." Or, "It will be all right, I'll make you some chocolate pudding." As he got older, it was, "Don't worry about it. Have an eclair."

What a terrible thing to do to children, to turn them into fatties by making everything revolve around food! You can teach a child to use food as a reward, as a solace, as the answer to everything.

Our younger son, Richard, who's now 15, was obviously a born civilian because he always preferred food like oranges. He didn't have to fight the battle against obesity. It seemed unbelievable to me that Marty and I could have produced a child who didn't like eclairs and whipped cream and who preferred oranges—but we did. Given time, I'm sure I could have taught him to like eclairs, but, fortunately for him, I became involved with Weight Watchers first. I never had to change Richard's eating habits. And David slimmed down before he became an adolescent.

With two small children, I had plenty to do, but I always found more. I became involved in anything that came my way. And whatever organization I got into, I usually ended up heading it. Often I'd wind up as the president because I was always looking for a place to talk. I love to talk. And, as president, I'd be standing behind the podium where people couldn't see all of me. I guess I felt that if you've got the gavel in your hand, you're not only half hidden but you're respected for what you say, not how you look.

Things were still tight, so Marty took a job as a private chauffeur to supplement his income from bus driving. When he'd saved a little extra, he bought me a mink stole. That was in 1957.

Well, there I was with a mink stole and no place to wear it. I looked for a luncheon to go to. Where else was I going to wear a mink stole? Certainly not to the supermarket.

I heard from a neighbor that the North Hills League for Retarded Children was holding a raffle-book luncheon, and that anybody who sold a book of raffle tickets could attend the luncheon at the Waldorf-Astoria Hotel in Manhattan. So I got a book and I sold all the tickets. Door-to-door, 50 cents a ticket. Then I went to the luncheon at the Waldorf, wearing my mink stole.

Frankly, I had never seen a retarded child. I never knew anybody who had one. But I was inspired by the speakers and I wanted to work for a good cause, to do something for somebody else, and I decided I would join the organization that day.

David and Richard were still small, Marty was working nights and we couldn't afford baby-sitters. One day I mentioned this to Gloria, the neighbor who was a member of the League. "I'd like to do something, but I can't attend meetings," I told her.

She said, "That's all right. Just do anything to raise money. It's a fund-raising organization and they need money."

My mother was active in a charitable organization in Brooklyn, so I called her to ask if she knew anything I could buy wholesale. I wanted something I could keep in the baby-carriage basket and sell to my neighbors when I was wheeling the children. I knew I could sell because I never had trouble with words. Mother found a lady who sold me plastic tablecloths for 60 cents, and I sold them for a dollar. That year, I raised a couple of hundred dollars for retarded children simply by selling tablecloths.

This was considered so unusual that the next year I was elected fund raiser for the Little Neck chapter of the organization. I gave another girl the tablecloths to sell. I organized bazaars and dances and rummage sales, and I looked for something I could do at home at night. I decided to sell theater tickets. I found that you could buy a block of seats in a theater and sell them for a dollar or two over the box-office price. Anything over the box-office price went to the charity.

I just picked up the Queens telephone directory and, starting with "A," called people on the phone. Strangers, people I'd never met before. I simply said, "I represent the North Hills League for Retarded Children. We're running a theater benefit and we're charging $6.60, a dollar over the box-office price." I'd give them the little résumé of the play which I got from the broker and I'd tell them exactly where their seats were.

I earned $1,600 for the League in one season.

After a while, I didn't need the phone book anymore. I had a whole list of prospective ticket purchasers. A woman would say, "Oh, of course we'll go. And would you call my friend? I'm sure she'd like to go, too." "Sure, who's your friend?" And I'd call her. Some people didn't like musicals, so I'd make an index card for them: "Smith—no musicals." Then, when I had tickets for a straight play, I'd call them.

Other people would say, "I'd love to go, but we can't afford it."

I'd say, "If you will pay it out 25 cents a week, I'll be glad to keep records. And I'll deliver the tickets to you." I had people going to the theater who never went before. On a quarter a week, they never felt it, but the record-keeping involved was unbelievable.

I raised so much money that I was elected fund raiser for the second year.

Once a month, the members of our chapter visited a hospital for retarded children. We did small things, like paint the nails of a little girl or color a book with a little boy, just to give them a feeling that someone cared about them.

That summer, the chapter established a day camp for retarded children, and we took turns driving them to the camp site. I had Wednesdays and it was my job to pick up three children and deliver them and take them home at night.

The third year I belonged to the League, I was elected president. It was one of the happiest moments of my life. There I was, standing behind a podium with a gavel in my hand. I was president for two years in a row.

I've always found that the more you do, the more you want to do. I became involved in the P.T.A. and volunteered to be a den mother for cub scouts. I knew very little about making airplanes with kids and all that, but I wanted to be active, so I did it. I've always wanted to do everything all at once; I could never stand feeling useless or idle. I've always been like a firecracker, exploding in a million directions. I even talk that way, going off on different tangents. I work that way—never quite finishing one thing before I start another. I used to clean house the same way. I'd walk into the kitchen determined I was going to clean the stove, and if I had to go into the bedroom for something, I'd notice the dust and I'd start dusting the dresser. And then, if I had to answer the telephone in the living room, I'd spot something in there that needed straightening. I'm just beginning to learn that I can't do *everything* I want to do and so I have to decide what's most important. I'm beginning to learn that I don't have to do everything myself, that I can divide up the responsibilities.

All the jobs I took on in those days were good training for what has happened since then. I still keep up with some of them. I never miss two functions of the North Hills League for Retarded Children: the yearly donor dinner and the annual raffle-book luncheon. I've even flown in from out of town to attend. And in May, 1968, I was invited to be the guest lecturer. I'd attended the Waldorf luncheon for 10 years and now I was to be the honored speaker before 500 women. I didn't know what to say; how could I tie in Weight Watchers, which had become my life's work, with retarded children?

So I thanked them for giving me the opportunity to develop some stage presence when I was president of our chapter and I told them it was the foundation of what I was doing now.

I think everything you do in life helps you—if you know how to file it away and pull it out when you need it. I think that every experience has its place in your life. Things that I did 10, 15 or 20 years ago are bearing fruit, just like being fat, and all the things I went through as a fat woman help me to help other people now. I know how fat people feel. It never occurred to me at the time that I would ever be telling a huge audience the story of wearing drapes as a costume, that the humiliation of *having* to wear drapes because nothing else would cover me up would one day do some good and be inspirational to others.

I was still fat when I was working for the League. I weighed over 200 pounds and wore a size-44 dress. Marty weighed 265. He never dieted, but he suffered, too. Every time I went on a diet, he would say, "Oh, no, not again." He hated the whole thing. Not so much because of the diet but because he had to live for three or four months with a "crazy woman." I became irritable, high-strung and cried for no reason at all. Even my son David was old enough to know when Mommy was on a diet.

Well, I had a right to be irritable—I was deprived! I was miserable on celery and carrot sticks and I wanted some chocolate-covered marshmallow cookies. If I hid some in the bathroom hamper (and why, I don't know—

because Marty would have been delighted if I'd gone off the diet and become "human" again) and sneaked a few now and then, I was even more miserable . . . for how was I *ever* going to become thin?

I had gone on and off so many diets that I almost decided to forget about the whole problem and just be fat without worrying about it. After all, it was a good life even with 214 pounds.

Chapter Eight

ONE SEPTEMBER AFTERNOON IN 1961, I was pushing my shopping cart in a supermarket in Little Neck when a girl I hardly knew came up to me.

"You look so *marvelous*," she said to me. "Did you have a good summer?"

And I said, "Of course, I had a good summer." I always did. Little Neck is a community on Long Island where there are lots of trucks in the summertime—ice cream trucks, pizza trucks, doughnut trucks, hero sandwich trucks—and every truck passed right in front of my house. If they passed by too fast, I'd run down the block after them. I always found a good reason to buy a little something—it was a very good summer.

"You look so marvelous," she said again. "When are you due?"

That really hurt. I didn't like that girl then and I don't now, but I've been grateful to her ever since. Most fat people need to be hurt badly before they do something about themselves. Being told by a doctor that you have high blood pressure or heart trouble because you're fat isn't enough. Looking in a mirror isn't enough because when you walk away from a mirror, you forget what you look like. You think, "How nice my eyes are," and you forget your hips are monstrous. Something's got to happen to demoralize you suddenly and completely before you see the light. Some people have told me that what finally moved them was the first time they stood up in a restaurant and the chair came up with them.

I've met women who can afford to go to a beauty shop and don't because in a beauty shop there are arms on the chairs. We live in a world where we're finding ways to get to outer space—we've reached the moon—but we've never done anything positive up till now for the woman who says, "I can't go to the beauty parlor because the chairs have arms." We obviously must develop beauty shops with wider chairs or do something for these women.

Sometimes it's a small thing that makes a person decide to take action, like a saleslady in a dress shop saying, "Don't worry, madam. We'll let out the side seams as far as they can go." Or perhaps you have to get out of the back seat of a two-door car and one person has to pull and another has to push. Or a big thing, like your child coming home from school one day and saying, "It's Open School Week next week. Please don't come."

So. That girl thought I was pregnant. I didn't know what to say. I walked the four blocks home from the supermarket and thought, "What do I do now? I'm so fat I look nine months pregnant." I'd exhausted every doctor in my neighborhood. I'd gone to New Jersey for new diet doctors because I'd already tried most of them in the New York area. I'd been on every diet there was and I was always successful. I always lost the weight, but I always gained it back.

In the back of my mind, there was a nagging. I knew there was something else to try. I remembered a clinic for the obese that I'd heard about at least 10 years before. But, you know, something has to make you very angry or ashamed enough to be able to say, "Okay, help me." I felt I was too intelligent to have somebody teach me how to eat and, in 1961, you didn't tell anybody that you were going somewhere to be taught what to eat and when to eat it. After all, you're living, you're raising children, you're supposed to know what to eat. Of course, I knew. I knew that a green pepper was better than a cupcake—there was no question in my mind about that. But there had to be a miracle that was going to make me look at a cupcake and say, "I hate it!" And that was what I was looking for, a miracle.

So I called that same day in September, 1961, and got an appointment for October. I went to the clinic and I didn't tell anybody. I'll never forget that day if I live to be 1,000, because it was horrible. I wore a big flaring coat—they were in style, fortunately—and I thought I was hiding my fat. I stood as tall as I could and I wore high heels and I wore big earrings. I took hours with my hair and my face, hoping that the people there would never look below my neck. And I went to the New York City Department of Health Obesity Clinic.

When I got to the receptionist's desk, I couldn't bring myself to say "obesity clinic." So I said to the girl, "Where's the nutrition clinic?" I figured if she pointed me there, I'd find the room I needed. They did have a nutrition clinic and they also had an obesity clinic. Obviously, I didn't look like I was lacking in nutrition, because—very loudly and very clearly—she said to me, "You want the obesity clinic! It's down the hall, third door on your right!"

I walked into a room where a group of overweight, seemingly angry, very quiet women had already gathered. I stood in the back of that room and I looked at them and I thought, "How could they ever have let themselves go like that?"

I sat down with them and nobody uttered a word. We waited together for the "miracle." We waited for the "magic." We waited for the "cure." I thought, "Maybe someone will come and throw a potion on me and I'll be thin."

Soon a *very* slender woman walked in. All I could think about right then was an ice cream soda. As soon as I got out of there, I decided, I would have an ice cream soda. I wasn't even particularly fond of ice cream sodas, but they're easy—you just sit in a corner and you eat them and you don't really have to work at it.

So this thin woman—I'll call her Miss Jones—started to talk and her opening line was, "Ladies, how do you feel when you look at a smorgasbord table?"

A woman near me turned to me, "I feel . . . like diving in. Don't *you?*" I thought, "Ah, a friend."

Then Miss Jones said, "When I look at a smorgasbord, I get sick to my stomach."

What she didn't know! She didn't know that if you felt lonely enough or worried enough or frustrated enough, or even like celebrating enough—and if it doesn't move, you could eat it. She didn't know that if you needed a jelly bean badly enough, you could go looking for it in your son's pants pockets. And even if it was covered with dirt and crayon, you could eat it. She knew nothing; *she* got sick to her stomach from food!

And I thought to myself, "This is not for me. I've got to quit this thing. I'll go home and I'll find another diet." How could *anyone* get sick to her stomach from looking at food? *No* food ever made me sick to my stomach—not then and not now. I still look at food and I am not sick. Today it's only a question of whether I can eat it or not: Will it put weight on me or won't it? But I love food. I've never looked at any food in my life that didn't produce some spark of love in me—whether it was in a magazine or on TV or on a table. I guess everyone in that room felt the same way, except the teacher. *She* got nauseous when she looked at food.

Then Miss Jones proceeded to talk to us one at a time. She said to me, "Mrs. Nidetch, you will weigh 142 pounds. You are 5 feet 7 inches tall, you have a medium frame and this is what you will weigh."

I'd had it. I said, "That's utterly ridiculous. I can't weigh 142 pounds. Obviously, you didn't measure me correctly. No doubt you didn't notice that I have big bones. I have a large frame. I have big feet. My fingers are long. I'm a big woman. If I could weigh *175,* I would be delighted."

She said, "You are not big-boned. You have a medium frame, and you should weigh 142." She was the teacher and I couldn't argue with her, but I thought she was ridiculous. I could never be 142. I figured if I hit 175, if I ever lasted that long, I'd settle for that.

Then she gave us a piece of paper that told us what to eat, and said, "You are not to question, you are not to judge, you are not to ask why. You are just to eat the foods listed on this paper."

I looked at the paper and realized that I already had that piece of paper at home. I'd seen that diet many years before. But I had never followed it. I judged it and I changed it. Not only did I have that piece of paper, I had thousands of pieces of papers just like it. I saved diets. I pasted them in albums. I saved them in shoe boxes ready to go into albums. I even labeled them: "Don't like." "Like." "Works." "Doesn't work." "Makes you constipated." "Gives you gas." Whatever. And I had an album of diets I wrote myself, good ones. I could take a piece of paper, like the one I was holding, and rewrite it to suit myself.

Why was I at that clinic? What could they do for me that I hadn't been able to do for myself all along? They even insisted on that paper that I eat breakfast, and I couldn't eat breakfast. Breakfast made me nauseous. I wasn't going to eat it. It never occurred to me that the reason I got nauseous was that I did a lot of eating at 3 A.M.

You see, when you eat at night, you don't have to be careful. A cold pork chop is great because it doesn't count. How could it possibly be fattening when it's cold and greasy? You don't even like it, you were going to throw it away tomorrow anyway. And you hardly ate at all that day. Here you are, in the middle of the night, standing in the kitchen all by yourself. Nobody need ever know that you're eating. It can't be fattening. And if you eat a hard piece of bread with it, that can't be fattening either, although it would have been in the morning when it was fresh. Did you ever eat a cold pork chop and a hard piece of bread at 3 in the morning? It's horrible. So it can't count. Cold baked beans are in the same category.

And I'll tell you another thing that isn't fattening—a piece of candy that you don't like. If you're offered some candy and you prefer the caramel, take the jelly.

I used to refuse a piece of candy from my hostess. Especially if she was thin. I didn't want her to think I ate candy. So I'd say, "No, thank you" and then, when she went out of the room to answer the telephone, I'd steal it. I'd open the box very quietly, take a piece of candy and eat it. The only problem was, how could I get it out of my teeth by the time she came back? I admit it's ridiculous to steal candy from a hostess who offered it to you to begin with. But I did it.

"I can't eat breakfast. Can I double up on lunch?" I asked Miss Jones. I didn't like bread. . . . I could live without bread. So, was I entitled to a corn muffin every other day? Milk? . . . I hadn't had milk since I was a child. . . . I'd give up the milk and then, on Saturdays, I'd have a malted. If I gave up six days of milk, why couldn't I have one malted? That way, I'd even be saving a couple of calories.

She very calmly explained that, because we were at a clinic that was open to the public, the waiting lists were filled with people who needed assistance. If, therefore, we did not abide by the rules and regulations set down for us, we could not remain as members of the obesity clinic. I must say that I didn't "approve" of the food, the clinic or the teacher, but the thought that I could be "terminated" from a free clinic was pretty horrible. I'm really not sure how they do discharge you because I didn't allow it to happen to me. It must be like flunking kindergarten or getting fired from your father's business. Besides, it was like the last stop.

I met women who were terminated and they were hysterical. They said, "Where do I go from here?" I didn't know what I would do either if this didn't work. It was the last thing I could think of. It was the end of the road. So I stuck with it. And that's where I discovered that I could eat and not gain weight. I learned that breakfast is an important meal. It had never occurred to me before, I was so busy adding and subtracting calories. I found that you can eat and satisfy your hunger—and still lose weight.

I decided that the only way not to be afraid of being a dropout was simply not to tell anyone I was going to the clinic. Then, no one would ever know if I quit or was terminated. I went, and I didn't even tell my mother about it.

I ate the prescribed breakfast every morning. And I ate lunch and I ate the dinner and I drank the miserable milk and I ate the bread. I gave up cake and pizza and ice cream for Miss Jones. I ate her vegetables and fish.

And I went back every week and I gave her two pounds every week for 10 weeks. The only problem was that she was not as thrilled with my two pounds as I was. She said to me, "You should lose more if you are following the diet. What are you doing wrong?"

I said, "I don't know. I don't cheat. I eat everything that's written here. Maybe your scale is wrong, because on my scale at home I saw more." (Lie number one.) "Maybe I'm retaining water." (Lie number two.) Let her prove I wasn't! And I would say, "I'm constipated." (Lie number three.) How could she deny this? Then I'd say, "I'm pre-menstrual." (Lie number four.)

Finally, she said, "Mrs. Nidetch, this is the fourth week in a row you've been pre-menstrual."

The truth was, I *had* been cheating. Only, I couldn't tell her. How can you tell another woman who gets sick to her stomach when she looks at food that you *have* to have cookies? How do you tell another adult that you can't give up such a ridiculous thing as cookies? I was giving up so much to please her. I gave up ice cream. I gave up cake. I gave up nuts. I gave up all the things I loved, except cookies.

I told myself I had to kick the cookies. Why should I be so dependent on a stupid box of cookies? I took them in my car when I went to visit my mother in Brooklyn. This was an emergency measure, in case there wasn't a store open when I got there.

When I ate cookies, it wasn't just a few cookies. I would eat two boxes. You *have* to eat two boxes. I bought the kind that has two boxes attached to each other, and you don't just eat one box and put the other away. You lie in bed and you keep thinking, "There's another box in there." You have to get out of bed and eat it. There are no two ways about it.

By this time, Marty and the children knew I was going to the clinic, so I took the cookies into the bathroom. There's something not nice about eating cookies in the bathroom and you can never really admit it to anybody. But the bathroom is really the only place that's private, it's the only place where nobody will walk in on you. So you lock the door and you stand there and you kill the cookies. You brush your teeth and then the only problem is, what are you going to do with the empty boxes? You hide them in the bottom of the hamper and wait till everybody leaves the house before you sneak them into the garbage can.

But nobody wants to admit she's a failure. I couldn't bring myself to admit the cookies. And especially not to that teacher. I really wanted to tell someone, but I couldn't tell *her*. And I couldn't tell the other women in the clinic because they weren't telling the truth either. Everybody in that room said she was water-retentive. Everybody in that room said she was constipated. Everybody in that room said she was not doing anything wrong. I thought to myself, "How is it possible that I am the only one who's doing something wrong?" It *wasn't* possible, but I didn't know it then.

In the 10th week, I couldn't even look at Miss Jones because I was ashamed. The problem was all the lying. I planned lies while I sat in the subway going to the clinic. I had to lie because I couldn't tell her about the cookies. Someone who had never been fat could never understand what I was going through.

Chapter Nine

IT GOT SO BAD THAT I just had to talk about it. One afternoon, I called six friends—six *fat* friends—and invited them to my house. I just wanted to be with people who would understand. I said, "Come on over and let's talk." I didn't call anyone who might be sensitive, only people to whom I could say, "I found a new diet. I'll tell you about it."

These were the women who were the jolly ones, the ones who told jokes about their size: "Oh, I'm so fat, I take up two chairs." Or, "When I take off my girdle, it's like an explosion."

Everyone I called came—maybe they thought I had new recipes. (One of these girls was Helen, who is now a Weight Watchers lecturer. I'd first met Helen in the waiting room of a doctor in Flushing who prescribed appetite suppressants. She and I got to talking and, after our visit to the doctor, we went to the delicatessen across the street for a corned beef sandwich and French fries.)

None of the women noticed my 20-pound loss. Nobody noticed what I had gone through for 10 weeks. But on the Sunday before this get-together, I'd been to visit my mother. When I walked in, all 194 pounds of me, Mother said, "It's enough already. I don't like your neck." To this day, I don't know what my mother didn't like about my neck. I guess she'd never seen it before because it had always had several extra chins in front of it. She said, "Maybe five more pounds. Then you'll be perfect."

I said to my friends, "Listen, I've been going to a clinic for 10 weeks and I've got an announcement to make. I lost 20 pounds."

Complete silence. Then someone said, "You don't look it," and they all agreed. You have to understand that fat women used to be very reluctant to tell another fat woman she'd done well at losing weight.

I decided to go straight ahead. "I'm only serving coffee this afternoon," I said. "No cake. No cookies. And you have to listen!" I told them every detail of what I had just gone through, the entire 10 weeks. And then I got to the cookies. Everybody agreed with me that I had a right to eat those cookies. There was nothing so terrible about that, I was losing two pounds a week, what was the matter with that?

I thought if I could get my friends to go along with me, to stick to the diet too, maybe we'd all be able to make it together. After all, for the first time in my life I wasn't grinding my teeth at night from taking pills, and my nails were growing. I wasn't losing two pounds plus every week, but I was losing two pounds. And I wasn't even hungry. I was eating three meals a day. The other girls could do it, too, if I could.

I needed the girls. I needed to be able to tell them about my difficulties. It was a selfish motive, I admit. I've found that all overweight people have this tremendous desire to talk. Maybe we're all "oral" types—we have to eat or talk. We have to talk about our problems and what we're trying to do about them. *Other* people aren't interested. Skinny people have so many other things to discuss and, if you persist, you're a bore.

There in that room, the six of us talked. Simply talked. I discovered that my friend Sue bought chocolate chip cookies for her children and kept them in the dish closet behind a platter. . . . Somebody else kept a can of nuts in a cupboard in back of two cans of asparagus. Obviously, her children would never move a can of asparagus in a million years. . . . We found that we all got up in the middle of the night to have a little snack. It wasn't Weight Watchers that day, it was six fat women listening to each other talk.

One girl said, "Jean, can we come back next week?"

I said, "Sure. Let's make it a weekly thing. Let's just talk. This new diet is working for me. I know we can lose weight if we want to. We'll talk about it and maybe together we can make it."

Was it possible for us to go to a movie and watch the picture—and not eat popcorn? Could we get up from the theater seat and go to the ladies' room—and not stop at

the candy counter? Were we capable of being at a party—
and not eating the foods we knew (nobody needed a
printed piece of paper to tell her) were fattening? Could
we do it? We decided to try.

Then I said, "Here's the diet I got at the clinic. Write
it down. And every one of you must promise me one
thing. Take it to your doctor right away. Ask him if it's
okay for you." This was important because I believe no one
should prescribe for anyone else. That can be dangerous,
taking diets from another woman. If you have a medical
question, you go to your doctor. We'd had examinations
at the clinic and I knew this diet worked for me, but I
didn't know if one of the girls was pregnant or if she had
an ulcer or a spastic stomach—maybe all the roughage in
the diet wouldn't be good. So, they all promised faithfully
that they would take it to their doctors and get approval,
and we would meet the following Wednesday.

And that's what happened. Except that on the following
Wednesday, the six girls brought three of their friends.
Three strangers to me, and unbelievably fat. The six
veterans from the week before talked. The three new ones
listened and tried to figure out what this whole thing was
all about.

One of the originals said a friend had visited her that past
Sunday and brought a cake. "But I sent the cake home with
her," she announced.

"Wasn't she insulted?" asked someone.

"No. I told her nobody in our house could eat that
flavor, it gave us hives. Anyway, she took it back home.
Even if she was insulted, I don't care. I wasn't going to
sleep with that cake in my house."

Everybody applauded.

"You know something?" she said, "I bet I didn't even
lose weight this week, even without the cake."

I said, "Okay. So you didn't lose weight. Plenty of people go through a red light without getting a ticket. That
doesn't make it okay to pass red lights. It means they were
lucky, that's all. It's like saying, 'I gave up the cake and
didn't lose weight, so why should I bother?' It doesn't mean
you weren't doing the right thing."

Then I said, "Let's stick with it one more week. Is anybody going to a party this weekend?"

Sally said that she was going to a wedding Saturday
night. "Okay," I told her, "call me Friday afternoon, And

if you have to, call me Saturday morning." Someone else said, "Call me, too."

It turned out that another girl was going to a party Saturday night, and another was going to the movies. I decided, "We'll meet again Saturday afternoon to give us another shot in the arm." So we met again, and on Saturday afternoon four more new women came. The group was getting bigger and we decided to keep going. We met on Wednesdays and Saturdays. Wednesday was the regular meeting, Saturday was to fortify us for the weekend.

We didn't have a name for the group. I was the leader simply because we were meeting in my house and, as usual, I did most of the talking. But everybody talked. As the weeks went on, the girls started to show how big their belts were getting on them, and how their zippers closed more easily. A girl would walk in and say, "This is a skirt I haven't worn since last year—I couldn't close it." That's the way we talked.

I remember one girl saying that she'd bought eclairs for the *children*, and everyone laughed. It was funny because it was something we'd all said. When you weigh 220 pounds and you have two skinny little kids like this woman had and you say you buy eclairs for the kids, well, that's a funny line. She wasn't even aware she was saying something funny.

As the laughter died down, she added in all seriousness, "I keep them in the oven."

Somebody said, "You're supposed to keep eclairs in the refrigerator."

I interrupted, "You keep them in the oven because nobody is going to look for them there. If your husband or one of your skinny kids decided to have one of those eclairs you bought for them, they'd never think to look in the oven. They'd look in the refrigerator. Then you have all those leftover eclairs in the oven and you can't throw them out, can you?" Then she laughed and admitted that there was some truth in this.

We had discovered something—we'd been kidding ourselves. I used to buy candy bars and freeze them. But I never put them in the front of the freezer. I very carefully put them behind something else. To put a box of candy in a freezer behind a five-pound roast beef takes a great deal of ingenuity. You have to think ahead: Should you not be home one night and should your youngster go looking for the candy that you conscientiously told him you bought for him, he wouldn't think to move the roast beef to find it. He'd open the door, look around, not see the candy and close the door again. And guess who would have the candy the next day?

Until I talked about it with those women, I never consciously realized that it wasn't accidental that the kids didn't eat the candy and I did.

Another woman told us she used to buy a cake for dessert. By the time dinner was served, she'd have eaten three-quarters of it. As a result, everybody else in the family got a sliver.

It was such a relief to be able to admit to other people that although you picked at your food all day, you got up in the middle of the night to eat cold baked beans, that you hid the eclairs in the oven and kept candy behind the roast beef in the freezer.

We not only kept discovering things about ourselves, but now, because we were confessing to the others, we could help ourselves stop doing what we knew we shouldn't be doing. Besides, we had fun.

Every week, more women came to our meetings. Within two months, there were 40 of us meeting at my house. They flowed over into the kitchen and they had to bring their own chairs. They had to sit in the bedroom and in the foyer. Everyone talked and the veterans stood up and said something encouraging to the new ones. Mostly, *I* talked—and talked—and talked.

I quit the clinic the second week of the meetings because I was able to derive from the meetings more than I'd been getting from the clinic. I never went back. I wasn't terminated, I just quit. I was still losing weight and I wasn't eating the cookies. I was losing more than two pounds every week. So you see, my thin teacher was right. I *was* capable of losing faster.

We all chipped in and bought a medical scale, which was kept in my house. Everybody weighed in every week, with one of the girls recording the weights.

We mimeographed the diet on a machine we borrowed, and I still insisted every new person who came to the meetings check it out with her doctor before starting. After a while, because it made me nervous of have so many people following a diet I had found, I typed up the following statement:

"I, the undersigned, am fully aware that Jean Nidetch is not a doctor or a nutritionist or a dietitian. I go to her meetings to be encouraged to avoid eating fattening foods. She has suggested that I see my own physician before embarking on this or any other method of losing weight."

I insisted that everyone who came to the meetings sign it. It probably was not a legal document because they signed it like a petition, one name after the other. Eventually there were hundreds of names on that paper because I kept it in a folder and, when somebody new came, I'd say, "I want you to read this, then please sign it." (Now, of course, every member of Weight Watchers signs a more professional version of that release. And in New York City, the law requires a doctor's approval before you can join a weight reduction organization; we are delighted. As a matter of fact, Al Lippert, who is now our chairman of the board, personally appeared before the Department of Health in support of this law.)

Soon there was no more space in my apartment; 40 women met there regularly and more were clamoring for admission. So I looked for a place which would accommodate all those people at one time. I found it—in the cellar of my apartment house. Calling it a basement would be very kind. The place was ugly. There were cement walls, tiny windows, no electrical outlets, a little door, pipes all over the ceiling and plenty of junk. I asked one of the porters in the neighborhood to clear it out. Then I put in a table, a wastebasket and the scale, and I bought a padlock for the door. I asked everyone who came to the meetings to bring a folding chair. I remember one woman who drove up in a chauffeur-driven car each week, stepped out in her mink coat and carried her bridge chair under her arm into the cellar.

During the winter, we had heaters running on batteries, and our lamp had to be connected with extension cords to an outlet in my apartment upstairs.

But people came, more and more people. At this point, I was holding two meetings a week: one on Wednesday afternoons and one on Saturday afternoons. The Saturday afternoon session was for the working people who couldn't come on Wednesday and for those who needed bolstering before going out Saturday night. This was the group that the men started to infiltrate. Here and there a brave man, the husband or brother of one of the women, would join the ladies.

People who had never before been able to stay on a diet were losing weight steadily. I'd say, "You've *got* to eat this way. I'm eating, I have plenty to eat, and I'm losing weight." I kept telling them that they *had* to stick to the program. They couldn't cheat. Nobody could be with them every minute to watch them.

One of the girls laughed one day when I said that. She told us that a few nights before, she had been so hungry that she'd gone to her refrigerator to see what she could find. As she opened the door, a fly buzzed around her head. She thought, "Oh, good Lord! It's Jean!" And she closed the door right up again.

We were all doing so well that we decided we needed a reward—everyone who loses weight wants recognition.

Someone said, "Let's all go out for dinner one night and eat everything we used to eat. We've all been so good for so long."

Someone else said, "I haven't eaten a corned beef club sandwich for a month!"

"No," I insisted, "the reward can't be food. We'll go to the theater."

"Okay, but where will we eat before the theater?"

That killed the theater idea.

Jewelry—that would be good. It was something we couldn't eat. "We'll all wear the same pin," I decided. "We'll have a pin made up with a '10' in the middle. We'll get the pins when we've lost 10 pounds. And for every 10 pounds over that, we'll add a little stone. How about that?"

Everyone thought it was a fine idea. So I called a jeweler and asked him to make up pins. The problem was, how to pay for them. I decided that everyone should chip in a quarter each per week until there was enough money to buy them (later we raised it to 50 cents). The jeweler designed a gold pin which cost $12.50. You really couldn't put a fake stone in real gold, so of course the stones had to be diamond chips. Each chip cost about $4.50. We decided that a person should attend meetings for at least 16 weeks before receiving the pin. That's four months. It takes about a month for a fat woman to accept the whole idea—she just doesn't believe it's going to work for her. Then, the second month, she rewrites the diet; she decides she can do it better. It's only in the third month that she really starts following the program faithfully, and by the fourth month, she's probably lost 10 pounds and is entitled to her reward.

We were all losing weight and we were having a lot of laughs besides. We'd celebrate once in a while by serving radish roses and green pepper strips. But I was getting busier and busier and Marty was complaining that my "little project" was getting out of hand. I had started getting phone calls from strangers—in the Bronx, in Brooklyn, on Long Island.

The calls went like this:

"Mrs. Nidetch, my cousin goes to your meetings. I live in the Bronx. I weigh 300 pounds and I can't get to your house. Can you come and talk to me?"

I'd say, "We meet on Wednesdays and Saturdays. Can't you come then?"

"But you don't understand," she'd say. "I weigh over 300 pounds and I don't go out of my house. I can't drive a car because I don't fit behind the wheel. My husband has left me. Sometimes I think I'm going to commit suicide."

Now, how do you listen to a story like that and hang up the phone and sleep at night? You just don't. So I'd say, "Well, all right, what's your address? I'll be there tomorrow." And I'd get in my car and go looking for the house in the Bronx. I'd find it and I'd ring the bell and a monstrous woman in a housedress, with unkempt hair and no make-up, would open the door. She wasn't kidding. She was always "over 300 pounds" because you don't say 380 when you weigh 380. You say, "I weigh over 300 pounds."

I was going wherever I was called, into the homes of women who were too fat or too sick or too ashamed to come to the meetings. I went everywhere like a gypsy, dragging the scale along in the back of my car. On Wednesdays and Saturdays, we were meeting in the cellar, but Monday, Tuesday, Thursday and Friday, I made house calls.

The first thing I'd ask when I arrived was: "Have you eaten lunch?"

The answer inevitably was: "No, I never eat lunch. I don't know why I'm fat. It must be glands." Sometimes they insisted, "It must be my metabolism."

And I'd say, "Do you have any tuna fish in the house, any eggs? You must eat lunch."

"But I can't eat and lose weight," the woman would say pathetically.

The most difficult thing in the world is to teach fat people to eat—not to *stop* eating, but to *start* eating the proper foods. You have to teach them to stay away from the wrong foods, to fill themselves up on the healthy foods so they won't be hungry.

Besides the house calls, these people as well as the women who came to the meetings often called me at home just to talk about their problems.

It was marvelous because people were losing weight and were so much happier. Finally I reached the goal that the nutritionist at the obesity clinic had suggested for me. She had been right. I *could* lose 72 pounds. I now wore a size 12 and I weighed a fantastic 142. The exact time I reached my goal was October 30, 1962, at 4 o'clock in the afternoon.

Marty, at this point, was not particularly intrigued with my success with this new project. In fact, he was rather distressed about the fact that we were no longer jolly eating partners and, besides, I was on the phone all the time. (He finally started on the program—and lost 70 pounds—but only after a bowling companion told him maybe his game would improve if he lost some weight. It did.)

My mother-in-law thought I'd be arrested. My own mother told me that the whole thing could never work for older people. Maybe it was fine for young women, but anyone past 60 would never go for it. It took a while, but I finally talked her into giving it a try. After she'd lost 57 pounds and went from a size 46 to a size 10, she admitted maybe I had something.

For me, everything was great. I loved what I was doing, but the meetings kept getting larger and soon I was about ready to drop from exhaustion. I couldn't stop. I had to keep going. But how could I do it all?

One day in June, 1962, I happened to be in a beauty parlor, sitting next to a woman who was telling her hairdresser that she was bored, that she had nothing to do all day.

I thought to myself, "Here I have two children, I do my own housework, I cook all the meals, I'm constantly running to my classes." I did all the weighing, kept all the records, did all the lecturing, and, in my free time, visited people or talked to them on the telephone.

If I knew someone had a birthday coming up, I'd call and say, "I am letting you know that you aren't going to eat cake just because it's your birthday." If I knew someone was going to a wedding, I'd call to warn her: "Don't you dare go within three feet of the hors d'oeuvres!"

As these things were going through my mind, I looked at the woman next to me in the beauty parlor and I wondered how anybody in this world could be bored.

So I turned to her and said, "Do you really want to do something?"

She answered, "I'd love to, but I don't know what. I've never *really* had a job."

I found myself saying to her, "Do you think you can operate a scale? If you can weigh people—and I'll show you how—can you be in my basement on Saturday afternoon? I can't pay you, but I'll give you something to do. I help people lose weight. I talk to them."

She didn't know anything about my little project, but she came to the cellar and helped me weigh in the people. The first week, I just said, "Thank you." The second week, I bought her a wallet because I was grateful for her help. By the third week, she became so involved with what we were doing and enjoyed it so much that she asked me whether she could help me on Wednesdays, too.

So, she became my first assistant. She's still with Weight Watchers today, but now she gets a salary. She's attractive and alive and involved with other people. She even lost 20 pounds. I hadn't realized she had a weight problem then because it wasn't obvious. How can you feel sympathy for someone who has the sniffles when you're lying in an oxygen tent with pneumonia? But she lost her 20 pounds and today she looks wonderful.

Chapter Ten

ONE DAY TOWARD the end of 1962, the phone rang. It was a woman who lived in Baldwin, Long Island. She said, "Mrs. Nidetch, my sister and her friends attend your classes and they are doing beautifully. My sister lost 35 pounds, and it's the first time she's ever got this far without giving up. I want to ask you something. There are 10 fat couples who all live in this same neighborhood in Baldwin. Do you think you could come and talk to us once a week about dieting?"

I decided to do it.

At first, I thought I was their entertainment on Friday nights. We met in their homes, and when I'd arrive dragging my scale, their children would announce, "Here comes the teacher!" Each person gave me $1 a week for my expenses. I was reluctant to take it, but, frankly, I needed it.

For four months I talked to this group. Everyone lost weight and we all became friends. At the end of the four months, I brought them their awards—the gold pins for the women and tie bars which I had designed for the men. I don't have to tell you that I was in debt at this point. For example, I had collected $1 a week for 16 weeks from a man in the Baldwin group who'd lost 65 pounds. I had to give him a tie bar, which cost $12.50 plus $4.50 for every chip. Each chip represented a 10-pound loss. No matter how you figured it, I was in the red.

I can't tell you why I gave the awards, except that when your child does something good, something you're proud of, you've got to reward him. And I think I was rewarding myself, too—it was exciting to be responsible for the success of so many people.

That night, in Baldwin, I presented the group with their gift-wrapped pins and tie bars, and the couple—Felice and

Al Lippert—at whose home the meeting was held that week asked me to stay for a talk after the meeting.

Al was a successful businessman and he couldn't understand why I was working so hard at my "little project."

"Look," he said to me, "my wife lost 50 pounds. I lost 40. Why do you feel you have to give *us* an obviously expensive gift? We should be buying *you* something."

"I don't know," I answered, "except that I'm thrilled to be able to give them to you. You all did so well."

Then he said, "This is ridiculous. It's got to stop. You're not a rich woman, are you? We're grateful to you for helping us lose weight and the best way we can show our appreciation is for me to give you some good, sound, business advice. First, I understand you do a lot of traveling."

He knew because I always told each group about the other people I was helping. It encouraged them.

He said, "You can't keep running around like this talking to people all over the place and not accepting money unless it's forced on you. You've got to form a business and let people come to *you*. They'll come because you seem to be able to get through to them. Look, I'm an intelligent man, but I was never able to lose weight before. Now, I've lost 40 pounds."

"But the diet is not new," I protested. "I didn't write it. It comes from the New York City Department of Health. I understand a Dr. Norman Jolliffe wrote it years ago."

"That's not the point," Al said. "You're the one who's making it work. You've really got something. But you can't operate this way. The first thing you have to do is stop giving out gold pins. The *pin* is significant and that's what makes it valuable, not the material it's made of. It could be made of lead and it wouldn't matter.

"Let me do something for you," he went on. "Why don't you see a jeweler I know and have a much less expensive pin and tie bar made up. Then let me help you incorporate, set up a business. You can rent some space so people can come to *you* and learn how to lose weight."

"I can't do that," I said. "This isn't a business. Besides, I couldn't pay another rent. Marty and I don't have any extra money."

"We'll work it out," Al said.

That was in April, 1963. By May 15th, I was a business called Weight Watchers.

We had to have a decent place to meet and it had to be

near where I lived. We found a loft in Little Neck. The landlord of the building took my mother, the Lipperts, Marty and me up to look at the space, the whole second floor over a movie house on Northern Boulevard. It was at night and it was dark and we wandered around the place with a flashlight.

At one time, the place had been used as a synagogue, with one tremendous room for that purpose and a smaller room for the Sunday school.

The landlord said, "If you are going to give talks to people, why don't you take the big room?" There was a platform at one end where the altar had been. "You could stand up here and talk." He wasn't at all sure what was going to go on up there, or even if he wanted to rent to us, but if we wanted to take the place, why not take all of it?

I said, "Oh, we couldn't. It's huge. What would I do with all that space?"

Without ever seeing the place in daylight, we rented the smaller room. Today, it's used for storage and we use the big one for classes. Sometimes I go back and sit in the little room and remember how it used to be in those early days. It seems like 1,000 years. That little room was IT— classroom, headquarters, everything. The rent was $75 a month including a new paint job and 50 folding chairs. A friend gave me a table and a desk.

The room was painted black. It had six or seven partitions. And one long wall. As the five of us stood there that night, looking around with the flashlight, we agreed that we would rip down the partitions and paint the place light green. But to myself, I thought, "Who will ever find me here . . . this room at the end of a hall, at the top of some stairs, over a movie house? Nobody will ever come here."

But they did come. Later, we moved our headquarters to Forest Hills, where we had five times the space, and then to Great Neck to our own building, but I don't ever want to give up that space in Little Neck.

I did give up the cellar. Some of the ladies who lived in Long Island were unhappy when we moved out of the cellar. They liked it there. They liked the way they could sneak into the meetings without anybody noticing them. In those days, people were ashamed to belong to a group such as this and they asked me not to have the name printed on the window of the new location.

Today, it's different. Today, at every Weight Watchers

office throughout the world, the name is displayed on the windows and doors, often in neon lights. Today, a member wears our pin or tie bar with pride and will usually tell you in a hurry what it means.

Two ladies I know met in Paris last summer. One was wearing the pin and the other wasn't. The non-pin wearer approached the pin wearer and said to her, "Are you from the States?"

The other one said, "Yes."

"Are you a Weight Watchers member?"

"Yes."

"Thank goodness! Let's have lunch together!"

The pin used to be like a hidden handshake. Now, everyone knows its meaning and we have buttons, bumper stickers, tags, pens, ash trays, many such items. We don't hide anymore. We've come a long way from the time when no one even wanted the name on the window.

At the beginning, we decided that we'd just tell people I'd already been seeing that we would be open and that they could come. Al felt, and still does, that word-of-mouth advertising is the best kind of promotion there is.

Well, on the morning of May 15th, there were about 200 people lined up outside the building. They came in cars, they came in buses, they came in taxis. When my assistant (the woman I'd met in the beauty parlor) and I saw the number of people who wanted to come in, we were astounded and frightened. I had never seen anything like it before. I wasn't prepared for a crowd—we couldn't even get them all into the place.

So, I finally announced to the people in line, "We'll take a group and I'll talk to them for about two hours. In two hours, another group can come back, and then two hours after that, the rest of you come back. While you're waiting, go home, go for coffee, go shopping."

It was unreal, but it happened. Most of these people were strangers to me, but all of them were overweight and they all had the same expression. It seems to me that all very overweight people look related to each other. They all look sad. They all have the same "wanting" look. It's a look of, "What can I do now? I can't think of anything else, so I've come to you." It's a crushed look, and they all have it, the very overweight. You see it in a youngster. You see it in an old person, everybody. That's what struck me when I looked at the crowd of people waiting to get inside that loft in Little Neck.

We asked people how they found out about us and they'd say, "Oh, my cousin told me about you." Or, "My neighbor's been coming to you."

On that very first day, I decided on an admission fee because I *did* have expenses. I had no idea what to charge, so Al and I discussed it. We decided that the movie downstairs had a $2 admission charge and if people figured $2 was the right price to see a movie, they certainly wouldn't object to paying that much if our meetings could help them lose weight. I had leaned toward charging only $1, but Al felt strongly about the $2, so we finally agreed that that would be the price.

I never thought about making a profit. I just wanted to pay our expenses. We had the rent, the telephone and electric bills, and we had to hire an accountant. After all, we were a business. And I had to pay my assistant to do the weighing.

We had built a little raised platform at one end of the long, narrow room because I wanted to be able to see everybody right down to the last row. On the platform was the small table that my friend had given to me instead of to the Salvation Army. On the table was a gavel; I used it to call the meeting to order.

I talked the way I always talk, and people listened. The beautiful thing was that they did listen. And every once in a while, someone in the group would stand up and say something.

A lady stood up at the very first meeting and said, "I'm a schoolteacher. I've been teaching school for many years, and I have a number of degrees. I have to tell you all something. Seven years ago, I watched a child throw away half a doughnut into the wastepaper basket. It happened at the end of the noon recess—and from noon until 3, I couldn't forget that there was half a doughnut lying in that wastebasket.

"When I dismissed the class at 3 o'clock, I closed the door and reached under the papers in the basket, took out the doughnut and ate it. The horrible thing about it is that it's troubled me for seven years. I'll never forget it, but I've never been able to tell anyone about it. Why did I do it? Just imagine what would have happened if someone had seen me! Just imagine if a child had come in and found me digging half a doughnut out of a wastepaper basket!"

At that moment, every single human being at the meeting was the schoolteacher's ally. Everyone in that room knew what she had gone through and how relieved she was to tell other people about it. And right then and there, I knew what Weight Watchers was all about.

Where are fat people going to tell their secrets? Most people really don't care. If you tell it to a size 7, she sits there and thinks, "Good grief, if you want to lose weight, why don't you stop eating? What's the big deal?" *She* can turn the whole thing on and off. *She* can stop eating. By her very expression, she is saying, "So, just don't eat!"

But you know something? You can't stop eating. That's as ridiculous as telling someone who's bleeding to death to stop bleeding. You can't.

Meanwhile, who can you tell? Who can you tell that you wake up in the middle of the night to go to the bathroom and you find yourself in the wrong room? Even if the bathroom is right next to your bedroom, somehow you manage to take the scenic route—via the refrigerator, where you stand eating something cold and tasteless, alone in the dark. Who can you tell that you can't leave any signs of your middle-of-the-night journey, that you have to make sure you don't leave any crumbs or a plate or anything else that will tell even your children that you did this terrible thing?

The next day, you're sure to tell someone that you never eat and you can't understand why you're fat. "I never eat lunch and my husband will tell you that I don't eat big dinners." That's true, but you forget to mention what happens in the middle of the night. It isn't even a pleasure because, when you get back to bed, you think to yourself, "I really didn't do it."

I recall a girl who told me that she got up one morning and she knew by what was *missing* from the refrigerator that she must have consumed a whole rye bread and two pounds of roast beef. She had bought the bread and the roast beef that day for a picnic—and it was gone in the morning. She had conveniently forgotten the whole experience.

Here, at Weight Watchers, you could talk. You could say, "I get up in the middle of the night and raid the refrigerator," and nobody would laugh—because so many people in the room did the same thing. You could say, "I hide in the bathroom and eat cookies because I'm afraid I'm going to get caught." You could tell the other people there that when you bought cake, you told somebody— probably the clerk in the bakery—that it was for the children. The clerk couldn't care less who it was for, but you simply had to tell her.

When everybody understands you, it's easy to talk. When I talked honestly to the people who came to my loft, they discovered that everybody had the same thoughts and experiences—and that made us all friends.

That first day in Little Neck, I felt guilty about accepting the $2 from those people. So I said to everyone at the end of each session, "For the same $2, you can come back every day this week if you like. You won't have to pay again." I wanted to give them more for their money than they would get for a $2 movie ticket.

And it's been that way ever since. I've always encouraged people to attend as many classes a week as they want, anywhere in the world where we have locations.

I kept individual records of every person in my classes. At the top of the paper, I wrote down the person's name, the date he joined, his starting weight, goal weight and any other pertinent information—especially his "Frankenstein." That's what I called the food he couldn't leave alone. Was it potato chips or peanuts or cookies or bread? I needed to know, because sometimes a person would come to class and say, "I don't know why I didn't lose weight this week," and I would usually discover it was because his Frankenstein had reared its ugly head. He had been cheating.

Another reason I needed to know was because, on the day a person reached his goal weight, I used to give him permission to eat the food that was forbidden on the Weight Watchers program. Whether it was pumpernickel bread, or candy or spaghetti with clam sauce, on that day I used to say, "Now, you can have it back."

What was so interesting was that often, when the person was given permission to have the food he wanted so desperately for so many months, he didn't want it anymore.

One night in Little Neck, a man came to my class and sat in the back row, where most newcomers would sit. I noticed him because he looked so angry. When the class was over, I couldn't resist saying to him, "Sir, does the Weight Watchers program make sense to you?"

And he said, "We'll see. I'll try it. I won't eat a loaf of bread at dinner anymore and I won't drink beer. But I'll never give up my doughnuts, not for you or anybody else." He spoke in a loud, angry voice.

I said, "That's fine with me, except that if you've got the courage to be here today, surely you've got the courage to follow the program. If you don't, I recommend that you don't continue coming here. Eat your doughnuts. Drink your beer. Nobody really cares. But if you really want to lose weight, there's only one way to do it. No doughnuts." Somehow, I knew the only way to get to him was to challenge him.

He was annoyed. The rest of the class sat there and smiled because they'd been through all of this before. I was a little worried. I thought perhaps I'd been too harsh with him.

But the next week, he came back. He was weighed in and, before the class began, I asked the weigher how he had done. She said he'd lost seven pounds. When it came time to call on him, as we call on everyone during the meeting unless they request that we do not, I said, "John, you've lost seven pounds this week."

He looked very proud and everyone applauded. I said, "Obviously, sir, you didn't eat any doughnuts."

Then he answered, angry again, "Not last week, but I am going to eat them this week."

I said, "That's entirely up to you."

And so we passed another week. He came back and he had lost more weight. I asked him about the doughnuts and again he threatened to eat some the coming week. But it was interesting to note that he moved up three rows. He no longer was sitting all the way in the back.

Every week, John lost weight and every week he threatened me with the doughnuts. Then the threat turned into a plea, "Jean, may I have just one?" He told us that before he had joined the class he used to buy a dozen doughnuts every night on his way home from work and he'd eat the entire dozen before dinner. It was a habit.

I told him, "John, you can't have it. Be patient, because later you can have your doughnuts back."

John finally lost 88 pounds and he could wear narrow pants and knit shirts, and he sat in the very front row, right in front of me. He became devoted to me and to the program, but he still had a loud, gruff voice. He gave

advice to all the newcomers and told anybody who talked
when I was speaking to be quiet and listen.

He looked great and he'd reached his goal weight, so
one night I said to him, "You know something, John?
You're thin now, you really don't need us anymore. Why
not come back once a month just to check in?

"And now," I added, "I want you to know you can have
your doughnut."

John stood up and turned to the class: "Ladies and
gentlemen," he intoned, "I've been a member of Weight
Watchers for seven and a half months. I've listened to
Jean give this advice to many people when they reached
their goal weight. I've heard her tell members they could
now have the thing they bargained for while they were on
the program. But I want you to know, I didn't wait for
her permission. Last night I went out and bought a dozen
doughnuts. All the way home, I was thinking, 'Now I'm
thin and I can have them.' I figured tonight was the night
she'd probably give me permission. But you know, a funny
thing happened—while I was busy losing weight, they
changed the recipe! Doughnuts don't taste so good anymore! I couldn't finish the first one."

The whole class realized that obviously nobody had
changed the recipe. But now, doughnuts meant something
entirely different to John. Now, they were frightening.
Doughnuts represented 88 pounds to him, and the fear of
being fat and angry and hurt and bewildered. I doubt that
John will ever eat a doughnut again without a funny
feeling.

I feel the same way about chocolate-covered marshmallow cookies. They're my Frankenstein. I tried them
recently, but do you know that they sort of stick in my
throat? They're delicious, but I'm afraid of them. They
represent size 44 to me. Now that I'm as thin as I want
to be, I occasionally eat potatoes, desserts, an extra piece
of bread. But I never eat chocolate-covered marshmallow
cookies.

Now that we were operating a business, I felt I must
constantly repeat that I was not a doctor and that members
must get their doctor's approval to join. I told them that I
had no way of knowing whether their particular bodies
could take this food. And I didn't want a person who lost
weight this way to feel, if she caught a cold, or developed
dandruff, or got a corn or a cavity, that she'd "lowered her

resistance" by giving up cake and candy. That gave her an excuse to go back to her old ways. I didn't want her to think that anything that happened had happened because of the program.

I have a tendency to develop little cysts on my eyelids and nobody has ever been able to discover why I get them. When I was fat, my mother used to say, "You know why you get these things? Because there's too much fat in your system."

I developed a cyst after losing 72 pounds and my mother said to me, "You know why you got that? Because you lost all that weight and you lowered your resistance." I adore my mother, but she's hardly a doctor. In fact, my doctor did say to me, after I'd lost my weight, "You've never been healthier."

I got colds when I was fat and I get colds now. I used to get a hangnail occasionally and I still do. I sneezed then and I sneeze now. Surely it can't be blamed on losing weight.

Occasionally, a doctor adjusts the diet slightly to accommodate a particular medical problem. Once in a while, a doctor will recommend that his patient not eat raw fruits and vegetables. Or that the person stay away from foods that produce gas. Or he should use no spices or salt. In such cases, the member must abide by his doctor's advice. That comes before *anything* we say.

If a person is allergic to fish, obviously he doesn't have to eat the fish, but we want the problem stated in writing from a doctor.

I remember a woman saying to me, "I have severe hay fever and the only thing that controls it is a lollipop."

I said to her, "If your doctor will put that in writing, I will be happy to allow you to have a lollipop."

She said, "Well, my doctor didn't really specify a lollipop. He said to keep my throat moist."

I answered, "May I suggest that you ask his opinion as to what can keep your throat moist other than a piece of candy?"

People come to us with the strangest arguments for special foods. One woman gained weight in our classes and blamed it on cough syrup. I found out it wasn't the cough syrup but, rather, the fact that she was eating cake. Because she wasn't feeling well, she felt she was entitled to eat what she wanted.

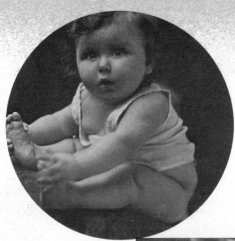

Jean as a nice chubby baby, 1924. It was cute to be a roly-poly.

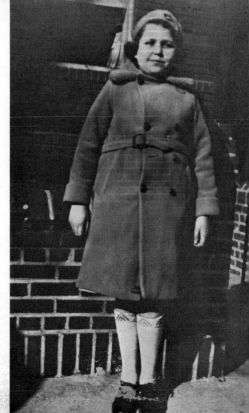

Jean, 9 years old, all bundled up for school.

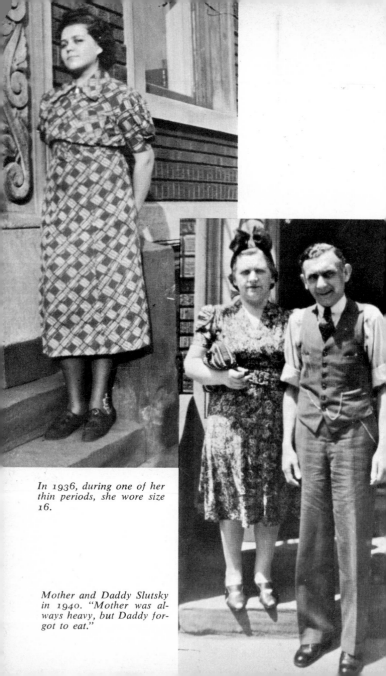

In 1936, during one of her thin periods, she wore size 16.

Mother and Daddy Slutsky in 1940. "Mother was always heavy, but Daddy forgot to eat."

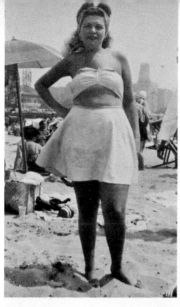

Jean as a bathing beauty in 1946, wearing a daring swimsuit.

Jean and Marty at their wedding in 1947. She wore a dress with an interesting neckline and a big beige cartwheel hat.

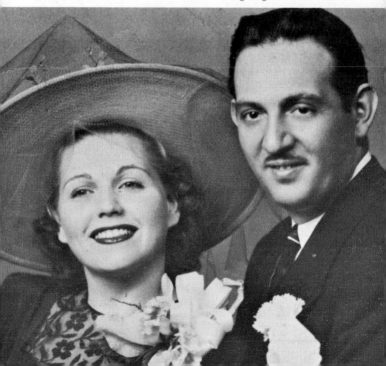

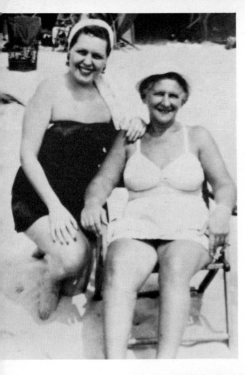

Jean and her mother at the beach in 1949, two cheerful fatties.

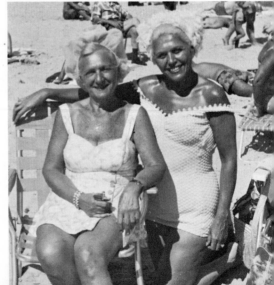

Jean and her mother at the beach in 1965, many pounds lighter.

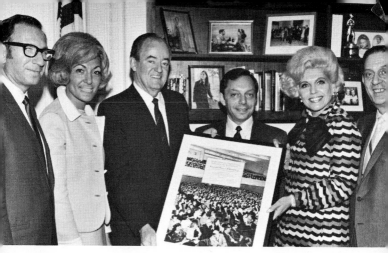

From left to right: Al and Felice Lippert, with then Vice-President Hubert Humphrey, New York Congressman Frank Brasco and Jean and Marty Nidetch.

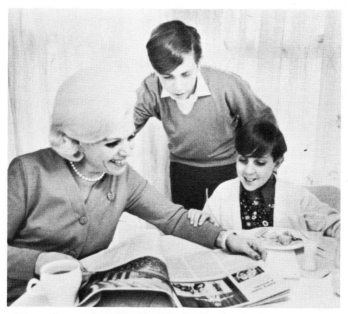

Jean and her two boys, David and Richard, in their kitchen in Little Neck, N.Y., look at a magazine article about Jean.

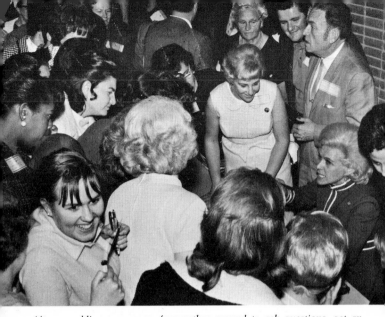

After a public appearance, fans gather around to ask questions, get an autograph, take a closer look or even touch her.

A class for members of a New York bank in 1968.

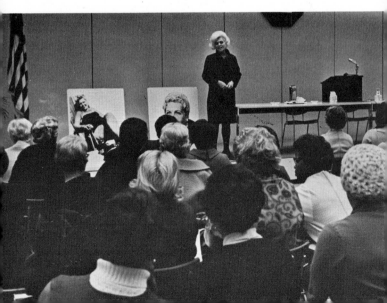

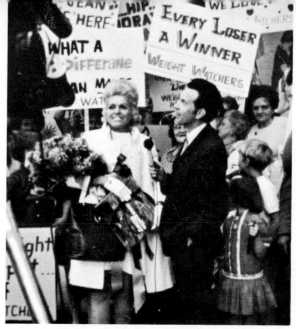

A welcome in Minneapolis. Jean arrives to a parade, a brass band and the television cameras before a public appearance.

On a visit to the Weight Watchers Ferosdel Camp for overweight girls.

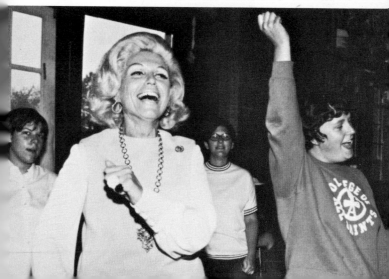

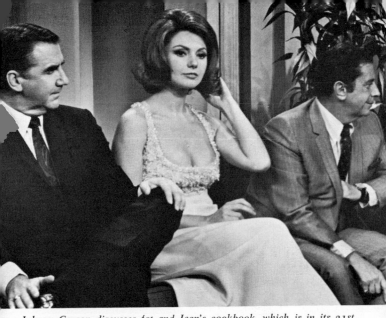

Johnny Carson discusses fat and Jean's cookbook, which is in its 21st printing. The others pictured are announcer Ed McMahon, actress Sylva Koseina and comic Morey Amsterdam.

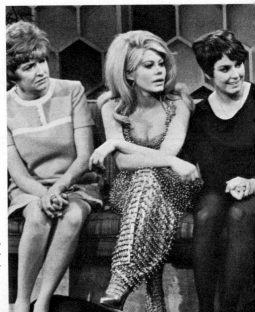

Jean appearing on "The Merv Griffin Show," one of the over 500 TV programs she's been on.

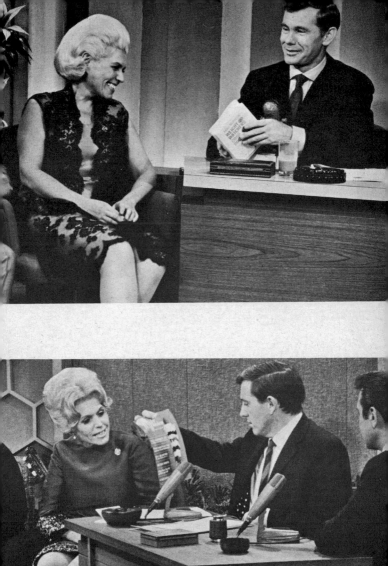
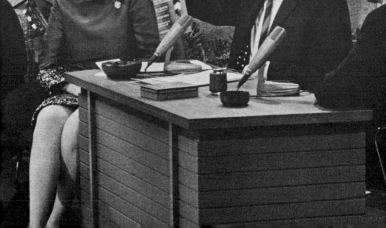

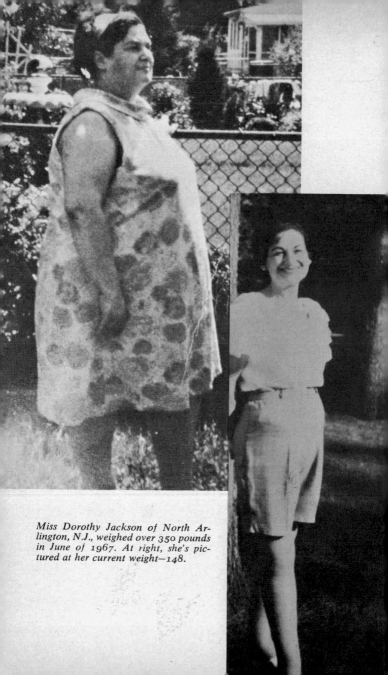

Miss Dorothy Jackson of North Arlington, N.J., weighed over 350 pounds in June of 1967. At right, she's pictured at her current weight—148.

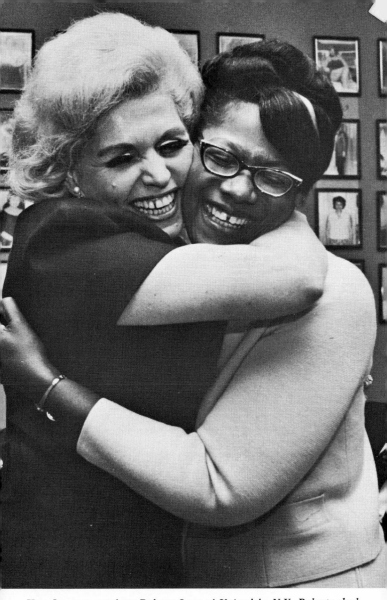

Here Jean congratulates Roberta Lans of Uniondale, N.Y. Roberta shed 90 pounds from a peak weight of 230.

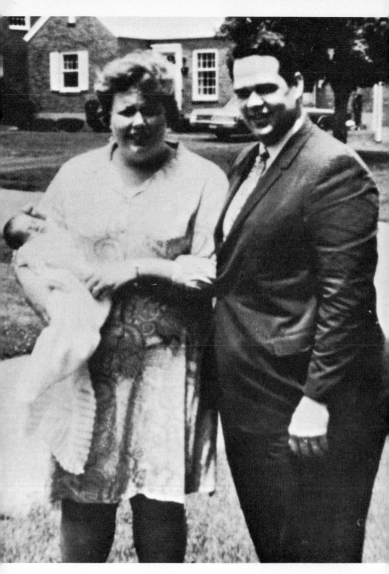

The handsome young couple pictured, right, are the same overweight two-some in the upper picture. Tom and Ann Mudd of Louisville, Ky., lost 125 and 119 pounds respectively, in the 12-month period between picture taking.

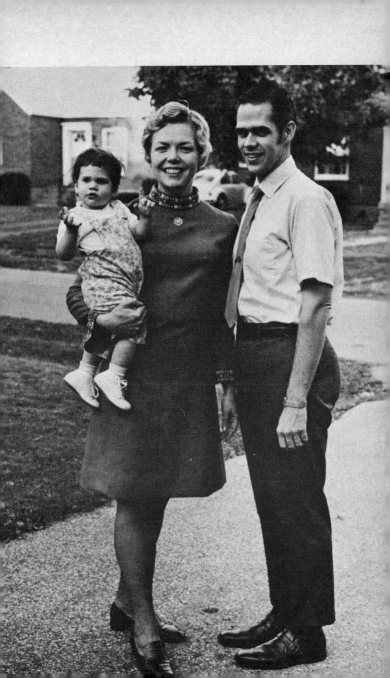

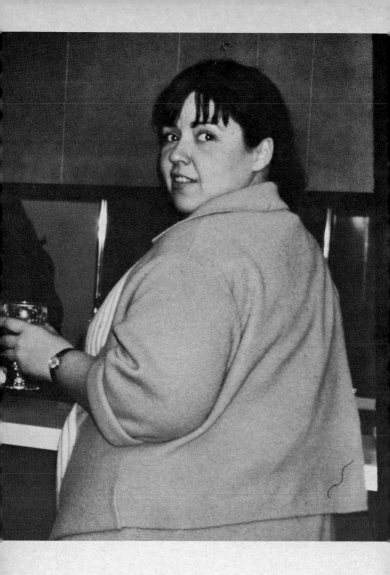

Nancy Blankenship, the pert young Louisville miss to the right, was once the 265-pound girl above. She lost nearly 110 pounds in a little more than a year.

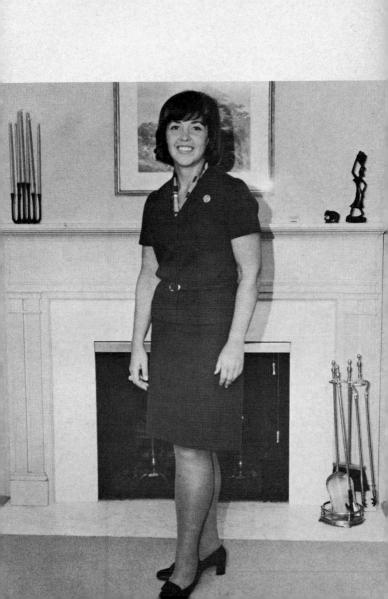

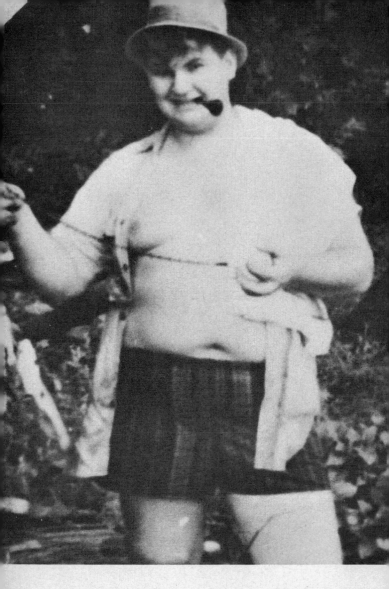

Lee Reed of Hampton, Va., weighed in at an even 300 pounds in July, 1964. He lost 138 pounds in less than 36 months and has since kept that weight loss.

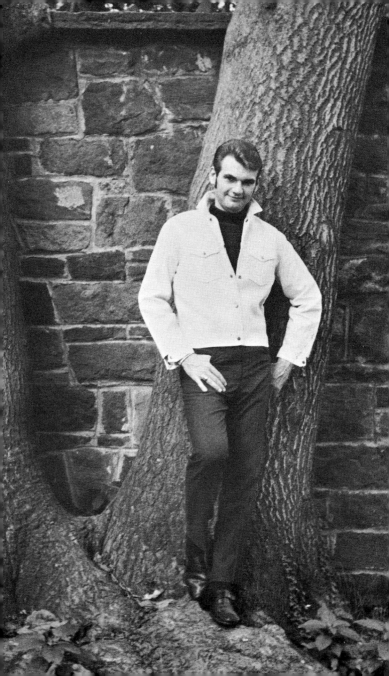

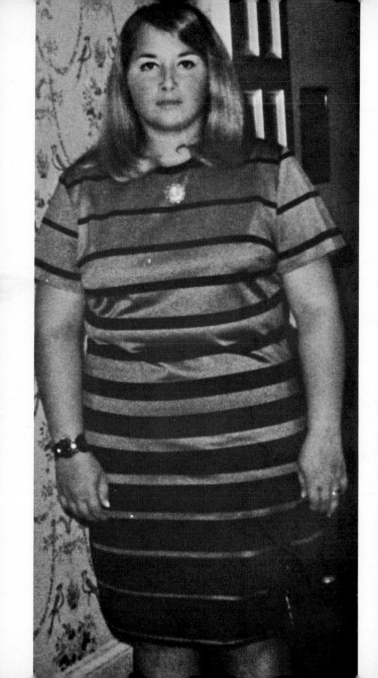

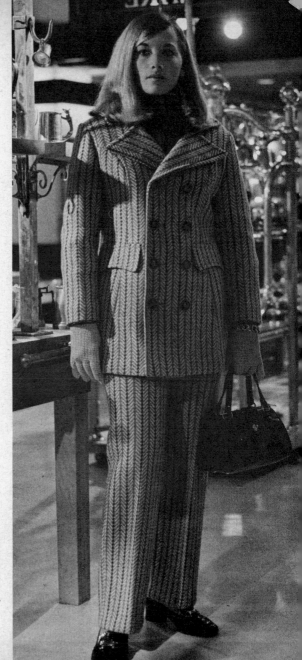

Randa Sale is now one of the prettiest girls at Washington University. The St. Louis miss lost 87 pounds from a top weight of 240.

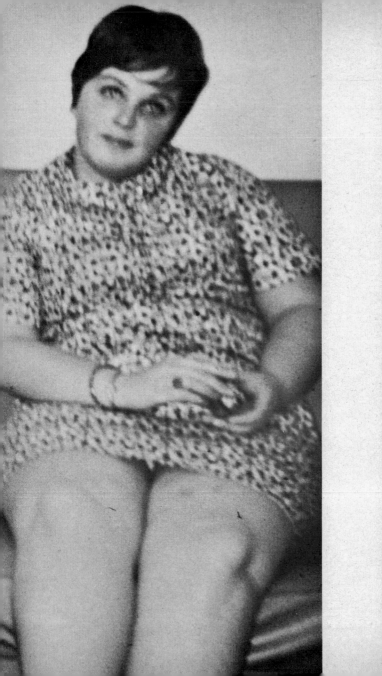

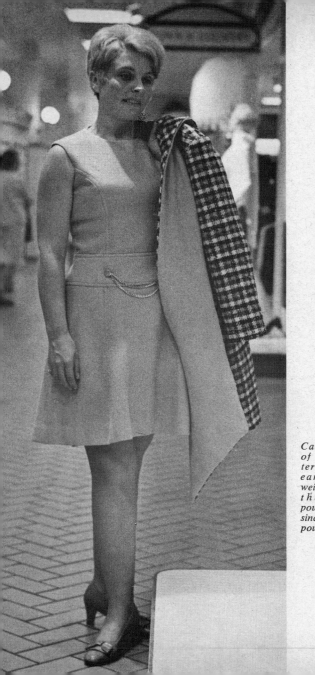

Carole Hart of Manchester, Mo., in early 1969 weighed more than 188 pounds. She's since lost 63 pounds.

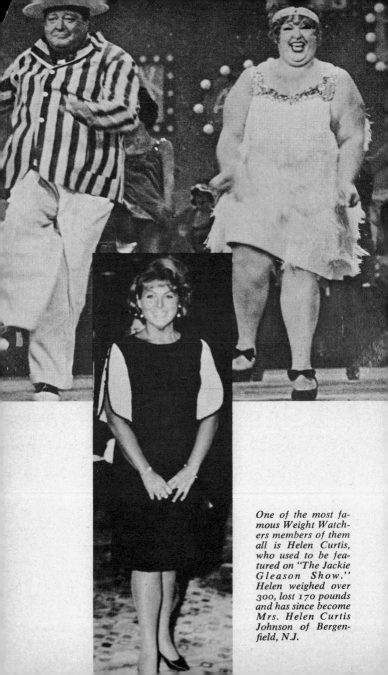

One of the most famous Weight Watchers members of them all is Helen Curtis, who used to be featured on "The Jackie Gleason Show." Helen weighed over 300, lost 170 pounds and has since become Mrs. Helen Curtis Johnson of Bergenfield, N.J.

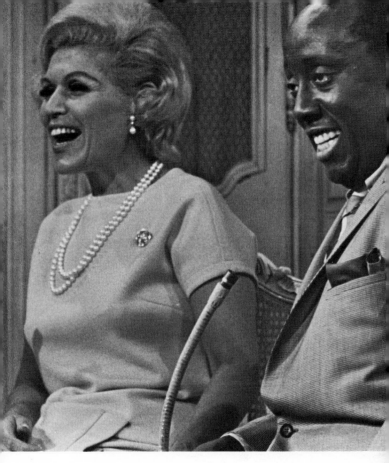

Jean with Godfrey Cambridge on "The Joan Rivers Show." Godfrey later went on to lose more than 100 pounds.

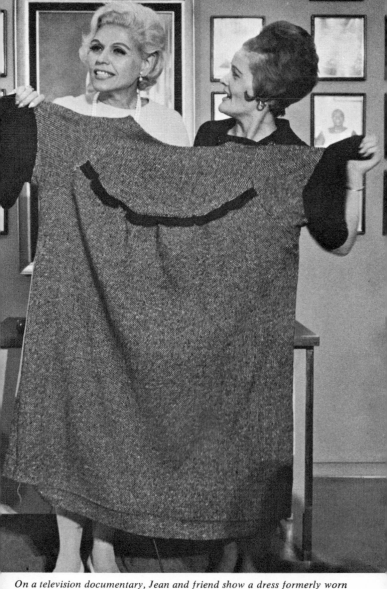

On a television documentary, Jean and friend show a dress formerly worn by a woman who lost over 200 pounds.

Here she's greeted by fans at the New Orleans airport.

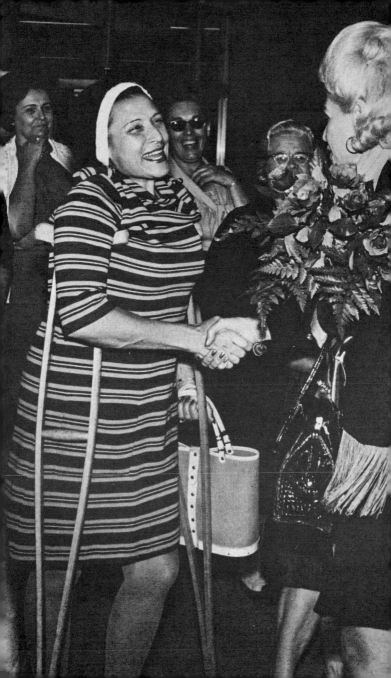

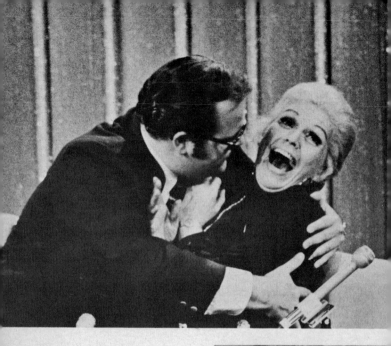

On television with another Weight Watchers member, Dom de Luise.

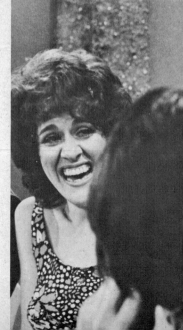

Jean with fellow Weight Watchers members Ruth Buzzi and Charles Nelson Reilly.

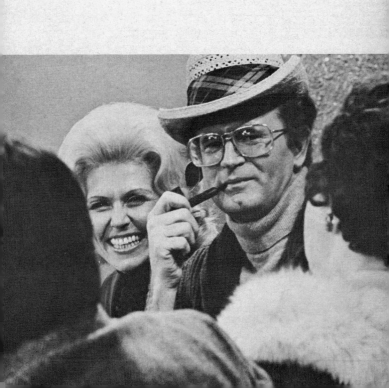

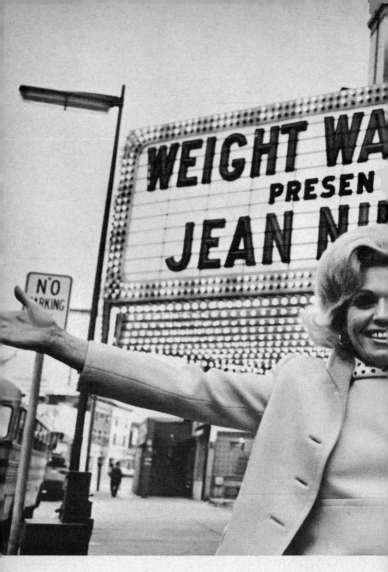

Minneapolis welcomes Jean and vice-versa.

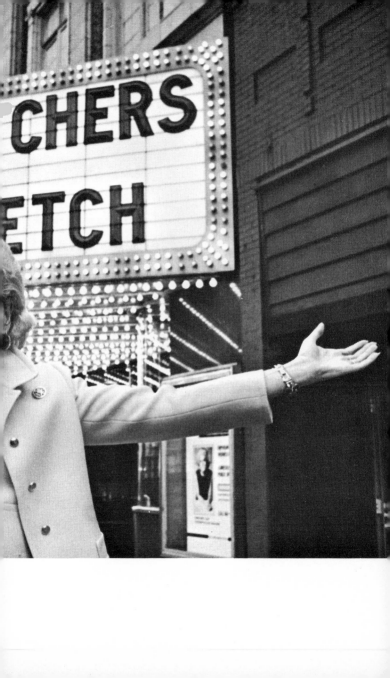

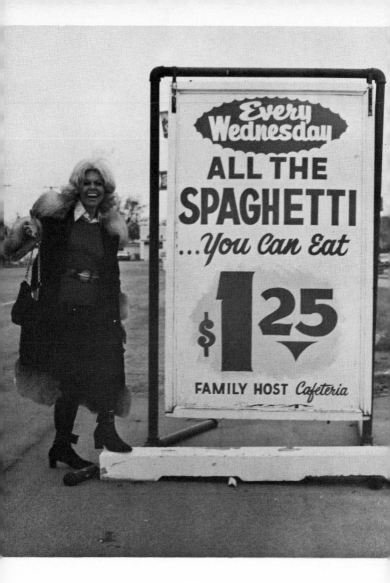

Now you can laugh at a sign like that.

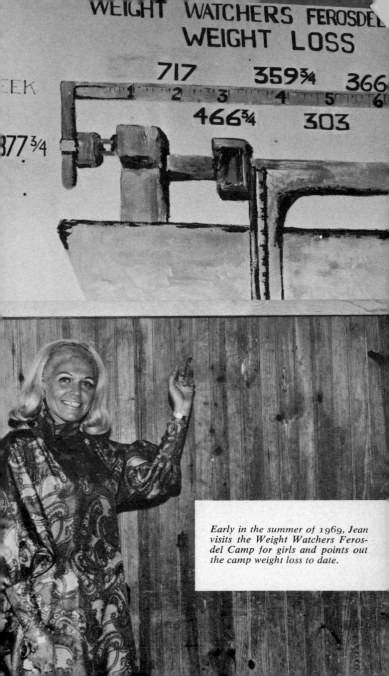

Early in the summer of 1969, Jean visits the Weight Watchers Ferosdel Camp for girls and points out the camp weight loss to date.

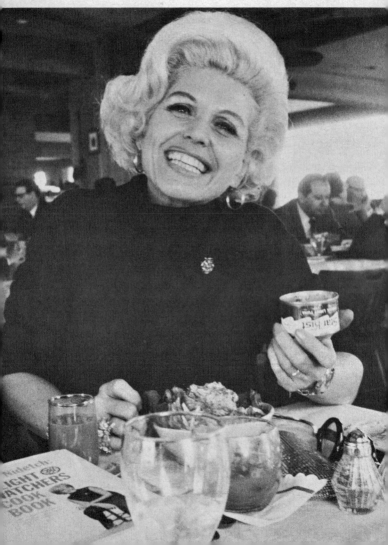

(Right) Just before going into the packed Academy of Music in Philadelphia. On the next two pages, you will see the inside scene. The few empty seats were later filled by Philadelphia lecturers.

Yes, she stays "legal." Here in a Louisville restaurant she digs into some tuna.

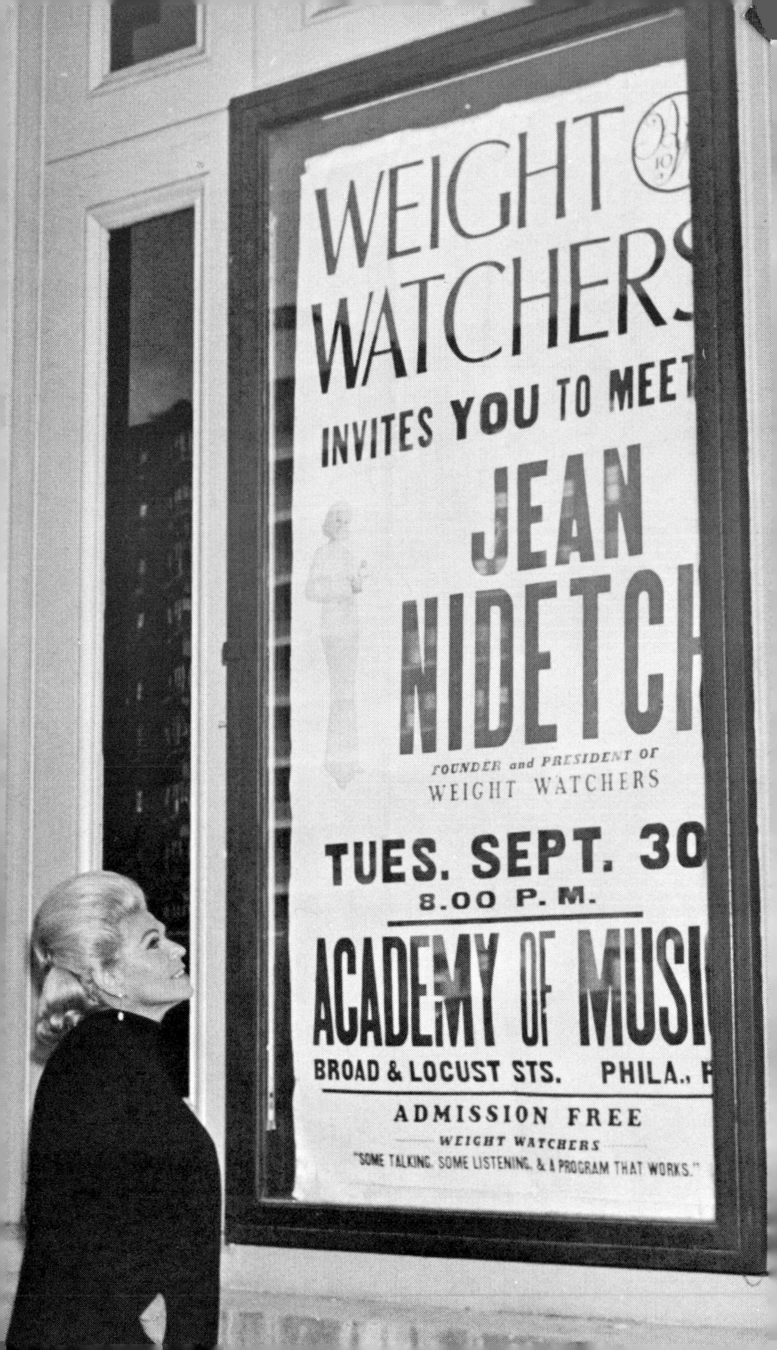

WEIGHT
WATCHERS
INVITES YOU TO MEET
JEAN
NIDETCH
FOUNDER and PRESIDENT OF
WEIGHT WATCHERS
TUES. SEPT. 30
8.00 P.M.
ACADEMY OF MUSI
BROAD & LOCUST STS. PHILA.,
ADMISSION FREE
WEIGHT WATCHERS
"SOME TALKING, SOME LISTENING, & A PROGRAM THAT WORKS."

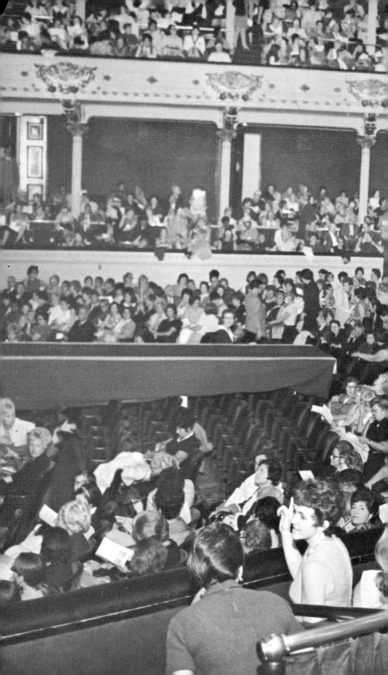

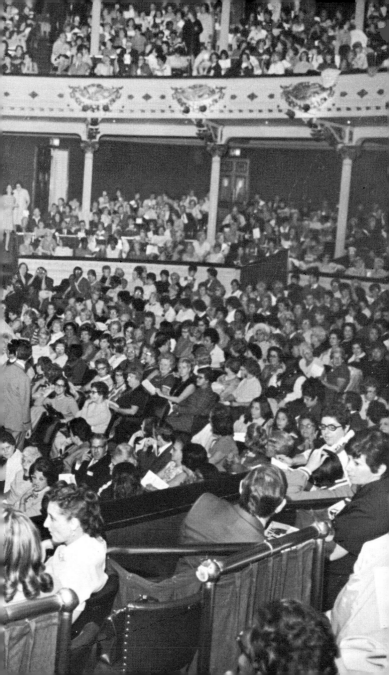

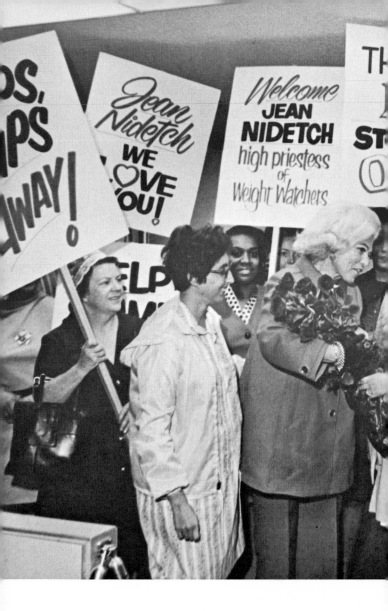

Another airport reception—this one in Washington, D.C.

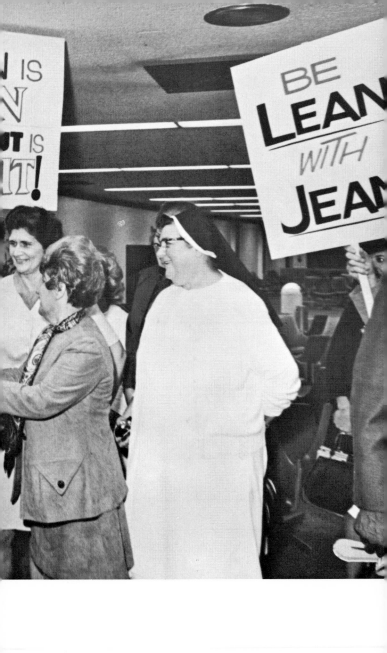

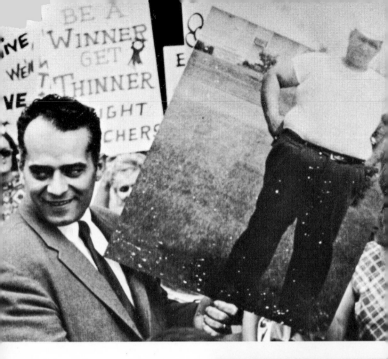

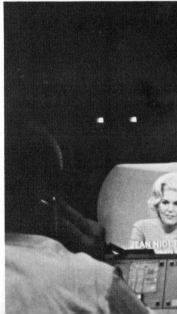

A TV director's eye view of Jean on camera.

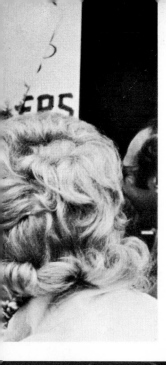

A more-than-100-pound loser greets Jean in Minneapolis with his "before" picture.

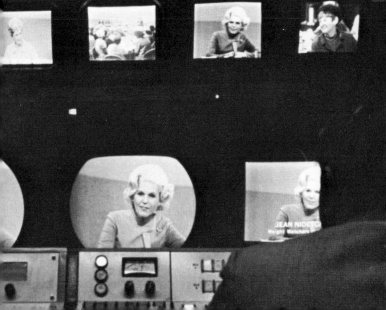

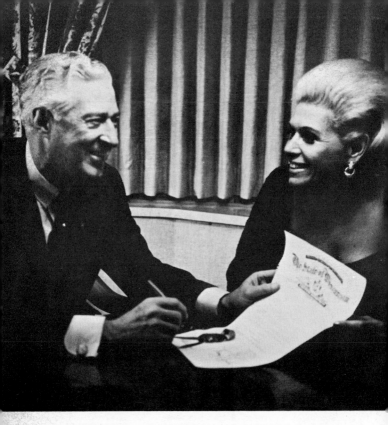

Governor Warren P. Knowles of Wisconsin proclaiming a Jean Nidetch Day and a Weight Watchers Week. Ceremonies such as this have taken place throughout the country.

I remember an elderly woman who said to me, "I've gained weight because of my grandchildren."

I said, "Are you sure it isn't because you're eating the wrong foods?"

"No, you really don't understand," she insisted. "When I look at my grandchildren, I gain weight."

I said, "Madam, unless you *eat* them, you're not going to gain weight from your grandchildren. Happiness is not fattening. Your grandchildren may make you deliriously happy, but obviously they are not responsible for your weight problem."

As the meeting was breaking up, the woman came over to me and whispered, "It's really pumpernickel and cream cheese." And at the next class, she admitted it to the entire group.

At first, I didn't know when to schedule classes, but then it occurred to me that you can't concentrate on disciplined eating when you have an empty stomach. I couldn't expect to make sense to a hungry person, because all he would be thinking about would be how soon he could get out of there and have something to eat. So, the meetings were scheduled at 10 in the morning, at 1 in the afternoon and at 8 at night, right after meals.

It was difficult getting the people not to come to meetings on empty stomachs. They thought they'd weigh less if they hadn't eaten for a few hours, but eventually they understood that that wasn't the important thing.

I'm sorry we have to use a scale—it's a real tyrant. But we must use it because there's no other yardstick. Often, a person who has been following the program diligently will get on the scale and find that he hasn't lost an ounce that week. And somebody who, a half hour before, has sneaked a chocolate bar, may have lost a pound. It's unfair. What we have to learn is that everything we eat, or don't eat, shows on the scale *eventually*.

I try to impress on people that a Weight Watchers member is really good only if she has survived a function where she and the buffet table were left all alone for 10 minutes and she didn't touch anything on it. That's the test, not what shows that very next time she gets up on the scale.

I went on with my daily routine of three classes a day, plus my weekly group in Baldwin, plus rushing home between classes to prepare dinner, clean the apartment and to market. My social life was dead. I got up very early every morning to get the boys off to school with their lunches and ran home in the afternoon to be there when they arrived.

After a while, I began to get hoarse from talking so much. I was tired. I decided I needed someone else to work with me and carry some of the load.

I approached one woman who had lost almost 50 pounds. She looked good and she was most enthusiastic about the program. I said to her, "Ruth, why don't you lecture? You can help other overweight people by telling them your own story of success."

She said, "I could never talk to fat people. I can't stand them."

I was shocked. "But how can you say that? I was here when you joined and you were *fat!*"

"No," she answered evenly, "I wasn't. I never was fat like *them*. I never looked like they do. I was just a little overweight."

That's when it dawned on me that people forget where they come from, or what they once were. It's like a rich woman who's forgotten she ever was poor and says things like, "How can you live with only one car?" Or "How can you get along without a cleaning lady?" It's like the girl who has her nose changed and forgets she was ever homely. Or the reformed smoker who can't tolerate other smokers.

We decided then that we would never let anyone work as a lecturer unless she'd been fat and remembered it very clearly. Not one person. We've had actresses come looking for employment saying they're between jobs, they've done parts, they've done Cleopatra, they can do anything. But you can't talk to fat people from a script. You can't memorize what you are going to say to this "professional" audience. You're not talking to novices. The people who come to us are professional dieters. They've lost weight many times and they know every trick in the book. Al Lippert, who selected and helped train the early lecturers, is particularly emphatic about this need for rapport with the members.

You can't stand up and recite a speech. You don't have to be a good speaker, you only have to be honest. So, when we look for lecturers, we find someone who wants to tell the world what's happened to her. We don't want anyone to lecture who never knew what it was to be fat and we don't want anyone who has forgotten what it was like. To help everyone remember, we insist each lecturer carry her own fat picture around with her.

As she lectures, a photograph of herself when she was fat is usually displayed right next to her. She knows she could easily look like that again and now the audience knows she has the very same problems they have.

Empathy is vital when you work with people. You don't have to be blind to work with the blind, but it's harder to understand blind people when you aren't. If you have experienced a big weight loss and the dignity it brings, if you can remember the feelings you had when you were fat and demoralized and if you can impart them to other people, you've got the perfect combination. It's obvious that you really are speaking from experience.

There was a girl in one of my classes who had lost 40 pounds and was really excited about Weight Watchers. After the class was over, I used to find her encouraging the newcomers. So I said, "Sue, why don't you work for me as a lecturer? If you can give me one night, maybe I'll be able to open a class in another area." She decided to do it because she enjoyed helping other people.

Soon after, a man called and said he'd heard of me from some friends. His wife had a weight problem but she didn't drive and couldn't come to Little Neck. If I would agree to help her, I could use his home to hold a class. Soon I was holding classes one afternoon a week and one night a week in Sheepshead Bay in Brooklyn. Meantime, I hired a clerk for the Little Neck office.

Before long, the groups were too large for the Brooklyn house, although it was a large one, and Marty and Al started looking for a loft, this time in a business area of Brooklyn. They found one on Kings Highway.

When I opened the Brooklyn and Baldwin offices, the very first piece of equipment I bought, even before a typewriter, was a red zipper pouch. That was because I was very superstitious. When I was collecting 25 cents for the pins each week in the cellar, the money was kept in a red pouch and it had, it seemed obvious to me, brought us all good fortune. The pouch, a pen, record cards and a scale were standard equipment for each office.

I made up my own system for keeping records. I had little index cards which I bought in the dime store and kept filed in a drawer. I didn't know any other way of doing it and it worked pretty well until Weight Watchers grew too complicated for my system.

For the members to keep, I designed a little report card to record their weights. "Weight Watchers" was printed at the top, and below it, my name and home phone number in case anyone needed assistance outside of class hours. And at the bottom, I printed a creed that I believe in. I didn't originate it, but I liked it and I adopted it. I don't know if anyone knows who wrote it originally, although I understand several other organizations use it, too.

It says: "May I be granted strength to accept the things I cannot change, the courage to change the things I can, and the wisdom to know the difference." It fit what we were doing perfectly.

The red pouch stayed with each office until one night, when there was a class in Baldwin, Al Lippert dropped in for a visit. He saw the pouch and he couldn't believe it.

He said to the clerk, "You have to get rid of that change purse and put in a cash box. It's not businesslike to collect money in that."

The next time I went to Baldwin, I didn't see the red pouch. I asked the clerk, "Where's the pouch?"

She answered, "Mr. Lippert was here and he said to use a cash box instead."

I shrieked, "We *have* to have the pouch! It's good luck! Where is it? Can you find it again?"

I was frantic. How could we *not* use the red zipper pouch?

I called Little Neck to find out if there had been instructions there about the pouch and, sure enough, Al had suggested changing to a cash box. I called him and we set up a meeting on the pouch situation.

I said to him, "You don't realize, we'll lose all our luck if we give up the red pouch."

"That's silly, Jean," he said. "This is a business now and you have to run it like a business."

It became a big issue and I wouldn't give in. Finally, Al said, "If you like a red pouch so much, why don't you frame one and have it hung in your office?"

And that's what I did. We used the cash boxes, but in my office in Little Neck, there was a red pouch in a frame on the wall.

For a long time, whenever a reporter would come up to interview me about Weight Watchers, I would tell the story of the red pouch because, in essence, it showed how a housewife's kaffee-klatsch became a big business.

Soon I was opening more classes. For a while, I held some in a member's house in the Bronx and then I found a room to rent in an office building on Burnside Avenue.

Each center had a telephone and was staffed by a Weight Watchers member who would take phone calls and accept new members. The classes grew quickly. A woman would call up one of our offices and say, "I'd like to come to your meetings. When do you have classes?"

The girl would answer, "We have classes on Mondays at 10, Wednesdays at 8 and Thursdays at 1."

Often the woman would say, "Oh, that's too bad. I'd like Tuesdays at 8."

The telephone girls were instructed to say, "May I have your name and address? As soon as we have a few more people who would like Tuesdays at 8, we'll open a class and let you know."

As soon as there were about 20 names on the list, we'd send out cards to announce a new class.

Chapter Eleven

MY LITTLE PROJECT was becoming a big, unwieldy business. I'd had no idea it would take off the way it did and I was getting confused and alarmed. Everybody was giving me suggestions: "Why don't you put up a big neon sign?" "Why don't you go public?" "Why don't you get a loudspeaker and broadcast your voice to the street?" "Wouldn't it be a good idea to appear in an auditorium?" "Maybe you ought to open classes in Westchester."

I was getting so mixed up and so tired of making all the decisions myself that I said to Marty, "It's crazy. The whole thing is getting out of hand, but you know I can't quit. Let's go talk to Al Lippert, maybe he can help me decide what to do now."

Al was involved in many businesses and I didn't really suspect that he would like to become involved with my project, but I knew he'd want to help me out. He was a dedicated member of Weight Watchers himself, he approved of what I was doing, we were friends and he'd been helping me make decisions regularly.

So Marty and I went to the Lipperts' home one night and I said to Al, "Listen, I don't know what it is I own here, but I want you to come in with me. I can't run it alone, and Marty hasn't had any business experience. Frankly, all I want to do is encourage people to lose weight. There must be some way for me to avoid having to make all the business decisions that seem to keep coming up. I want you to be part of 'this thing,' whatever it is."

Al decided to do it, and he and his wife, Felice, and Marty and I became partners. Al didn't give up his job and he could only help out part-time; Marty continued to drive the bus; Felice kept on with her chores at home. However, they were advising me and we met every Friday night at the Lipperts' home to discuss the problems that came up. And I don't think there was an evening that we weren't talking on the telephone. We made all our decisions together. We'll open a class in Flatbush. . . . Maybe we should think about an extra group in the Bronx. . . . How should we train the lecturers? . . . Should we give the clerks a raise? . . . What about insurance?

The Little Neck loft over the movie house soon became much too crowded and uncomfortable because our administrative staff was growing and so was our membership. My desk was in the back of the small room and I worked between classes answering the mail, which arrived by the bagful. I hired a secretary who worked at the same desk.

In one corner of the room was a tiny enclosure, no bigger than a small bathroom, which housed the scale. It cut into our space, but it was something I insisted on. At the obesity clinic, the weighing had been a horrible experience for me. It was done publicly in the outer room in front of everybody. There is nothing more cruel than insisting a fat person show, in public, how much he weighs. So we closed in the scale with partitions so each member could be weighed in private by a sympathetic, formerly fat weigher.

There was no way to expand in that loft because all the rest of the space in the building was rented. An art school had moved into the big room we hadn't taken and, between the school and us and the movie house, there was a lot of traffic in that small building.

Meanwhile, a little pizza restaurant had opened up downstairs next to the movie. The young owner, Romeo, realized within a short time that hundreds of people who came down from our loft passed up his pizza place. He couldn't understand it. Then he investigated, found out why—and made a brilliant move. With our written approval, he put a sign in his window: "We sell the 'Weight Watchers Shake.' " This was a shake we'd created, made with skim milk and frozen strawberries or instant coffee or vanilla extract, and recommended to our members as a pleasant way to meet their daily milk requirement. Romeo's business picked up immediately.

Then, with our approval, he put the "Weight Watchers Baked Apple" on his menu. Later, he began to serve other dishes made from the recipes we were passing around in class. Soon, Romeo no longer had a traditional pizza parlor

. . . he had added a Weight Watchers menu. He even put my picture in the window and I made him an honorary member. He became a watchdog for us. He wouldn't allow our members to eat anything "illegal" and he was tough about it. He served regular Italian food to civilians, but if you went in there wearing your Weight Watchers pin and tried to cheat, he wouldn't let you.

Like Topsy, Weight Watchers just kept on growing. It just grew of its own momentum. Obviously, we were giving people something they wanted.

We decided we needed larger quarters, and Manny Mark, our part-time accountant, suggested that we find new headquarters in Forest Hills. "Forest Hills is much more convenient than Little Neck for most people," he said. We agreed and he found a tremendous loft over a bank on Queens Boulevard. He was right. It was more accessible, there was a subway stop on the corner and a parking lot in the back. We moved there toward the end of 1964.

At first, we took just part of the loft because I couldn't believe we'd ever need the whole thing, and every year since, we've broken through the walls and become larger. The landlord built partitions for us so we could separate the meeting room from the weighing room and the office, which was just a small area with two desks, one for the Nidetches and one for the Lipperts.

Once-a-week meetings for the four of us were not enough to deal with all our problems, so we decided to meet more often. We were getting an enormous amount of mail with new proposals every day. One idea that came up regularly was to open Weight Watchers locations in other parts of the country.

Our first franchise was in Providence, R.I., and it was opened by Felice Lippert's sister, Elaine Robin. Felice lost 50 pounds in my classes, now wore a size 10 and, naturally, she told her sister about it. Elaine had had a weight problem all her life, so she rounded up two of her friends and the three of them drove down from Providence to Little Neck every week for 16 weeks, all losing weight successfully. Elaine had studied nutrition in college, had been a schoolteacher, spoke well and, after losing weight, looked marvelous. We decided to make a test—we would open Weight Watchers in Providence. We'd see how it worked out and then we'd consider other areas.

It was an immediate success. Since then, the number of

franchises has grown to over 100, and they're located in 49 states, Puerto Rico, eight provinces of Canada, and in England, Scotland, and Australia. All told, there are more than 21,000 classes a month. We also operate classes in West Germany and South Africa—and we've had inquiries from just about every country in the world, even from behind the Iron Curtain.

We've never solicited franchises. Most of them have been organized by people who succeeded in losing weight with us and then became interested in furthering the idea in other places. If someone in a distant city wants to open up a franchise, he must have a weight problem, he must lose weight on our program and come to New York to go through our training workshop before he may open. Most important, he has to be the right kind of person for the job, with sympathy and personality and a desire to help. Naturally, it is always recommended that the lecturers and the rest of the staff be formerly fat and have lost weight our way. For the most part, at our insistence, the Weight Watchers classes are the same all over, right down to the methods by which lecturers are evaluated.

Our training program is known as the "workshop." When we began to need more and more lecturers, we had to develop some efficient way to train them. I could no longer do it myself one by one as I had been doing.

Any Weight Watchers member, man or woman, who is five pounds from goal weight may apply to become a lecturer. We don't worry about age or even appearance. We worry about what's inside. A lecturer has to be able, first of all, to remember what it was like to be fat. If she's forgotten, she's not for us. She has to remember how she felt when she joined us, and she has to remember the feeling of dignity she developed as she lost weight. She must have compassion for other people's problems and, of course, she must have charm so her audience will respond to her. Learning how to interpret the program is the simplest part.

A lecturer must be able to talk easily and gracefully. Some people can do it and others can't. Our program is constant repetition of the same points and the lecturer has to get them across over and over again, making them interesting and convincing each time. The important thing is to be honest, to be yourself. Then you will reach people.

In the workshop, potential lecturers learn how to run a

class. Each one of them has a good idea already, having been a member, but there are things to learn. And not everyone makes it. The workshop training runs for nine weeks in three-week stages. Each person is evaluated by our training director (yes, that's something new!) and her assistants, as well as by veteran lecturers whose classes the trainees visit.

The danger in choosing lecturers and franchisees is that you might put people in charge who haven't got compassion. It's not like running an ice cream parlor. I know that if Weight Watchers didn't exist, I would be talking to overweight people somewhere. Maybe in my kitchen, or to a little group at a luncheon, or in the supermarket in front of the bread counter. The feeling has to be there. If you can turn that feeling into a profit-making commercial organization, that's a bonus. If you are a lifeguard and you dive in and pull someone out of the water, the fact that he may send you a reward later doesn't enter your mind at the moment you are saving him. You don't look in his wallet first, you just go out and save him.

Once a person has become a lecturer, she must weigh in every month. After all, we can't have fat people talking to a group about losing weight. She must not gain more than two pounds over her goal.

In February, 1967, Al Lippert came with us full time, and that is when Weight Watchers really began to grow into this big, successful, international organization that I find so hard to believe. Now he had time to run the business, plan our expansion and find the proper people to add to the staff. Frankly, it was amazing to all of us that this had to happen. But, with potential franchisees pounding on our door, and new centers and meeting places being opened all over Metropolitan New York, Al's presence was a necessity.

In September, 1968, we became a publicly held corporation with 1,025,000 shares outstanding. The stock opened at $11.25, peaked to $67 and has since split.

By 1968, even the Forest Hills space had become too small. We moved headquarters again, keeping Forest Hills for classes and the workshop. This time, we found our very own building in Great Neck, on Long Island, and it's had to be enlarged already. Here we have only the administrative offices and not even all of those. I've opened my own office in Manhattan because that's where most of my work is centered now. Al's coming into the business full time gave me more time to pursue my own special interest, really the only part of the whole thing that intrigues me— reaching overweight people personally. I want to reach every obese person in existence, to help them learn to live like human beings.

I travel all over the country and to our locations overseas, and I talk. I talk to huge audiences. I give newspaper and magazine interviews by the hundreds. I am constantly appearing on TV and radio—I've been on more than a thousand shows in the last five years, more than many real TV performers. There isn't a talk program I haven't been on, *The Merv Griffin Show*, the *Tonight Show*, the *Today Show*, all of them. And I love it.

I love to talk. I talk the way I used to eat—compulsively. And I like best to talk to people who aren't quite convinced about Weight Watchers yet. I can almost tell you the moment an audience begins to believe me. Whether or not they like me doesn't matter. I just want them to believe I was fat and now I'm not and the same thing can happen to them. I want them to know they're sitting there listening to me because they are unhappy and they want to change.

Quite unintentionally, and certainly more because of Al than me, Weight Watchers became more than just a way to lose weight. Helping people to lose is still, of course, the main object, but without our even looking for it, other business ventures started coming our way.

Aside from our franchise operation, for example, we have gone into the scale business. The program demands that the food be weighed and so we have always suggested that each member get a scale. Because some people had a problem finding them, Al arranged for us to buy scales in large lots from a manufacturer and sell them to members. Because we were unknown, he made arrangements for them to be shipped C.O.D., and even then the manufacturer agreed to ship them only because of a recommendation from a personal friend of Al.

Before long, the manufacturer said to us, "You're the largest user of postal scales in the country, so we would like to change the label from 'U.S. Postal Scale' to 'Weight Watchers Scale.'" Today, we order the scales in quantities of half a million at a time.

Everybody knows by this time that we are in the frozen

food business. It was a natural development because we knew how hard it sometimes is to cook yourself dinner when you get home after a day's work, especially when you must have a certain prescribed amount and prepare it in a certain way.

We market several prepared meals, all good-tasting, all wholesome food, all completely "legal," and all ready to pop into the oven as easily as we once grabbed a doughnut. We have four fish meals—ocean perch, haddock, sole and flounder, served with vegetables. We also have turkey, and we plan more.

We've found that not only the weight-conscious buy our frozen dinners but the general public as well because they get a good, hearty, substantial meal—bigger than the usual frozen TV dinner—and it tastes good, too.

My picture is on the frozen food boxes, standing there in a long white evening gown and holding a rose. It's really funny to find myself on a fish box, but I'm flattered and so is my mother.

My mother tells everybody in her supermarket, "That's my daughter."

I've told her, "Mother, you must stop doing that. Nobody believes you, anyway. Nobody's daughter is on a fish box."

The company has also arranged for the distribution of various other foods for the overweight sold under our trademark, including non-fat dry milk and a sugar substitute.

We have already opened a summer camp for overweight girls in West Copake, N.Y. In its first year, 146 girls lost a total of 3,091½ pounds while living a normal camp life and learning how to eat properly at the same time. We plan more camps, for boys and for adults, too.

I wish I could keep up with all the progress my "little club" has been making—there are even more projects in the wind—but I concentrate primarily on communicating with fat people. One way I do it is through the *Weight Watchers Magazine,* which is read by millions of people each month. In my "Ask Jean Nidetch" column, I answer questions from readers.

And my *Weight Watchers Cook Book* is now in its 21st printing.

There are hundreds of groups imitating us. It's flattering because nobody imitates a failure.

It really doesn't matter to me that these imitations exist. I just hope they copy us closely enough so the public isn't fooled and doesn't get discouraged if they join a quack group. Most of the imitation groups were started by former Weight Watchers members or their relatives. They just changed the name and copied everything else. They tell the Weight Watchers story, give *our* lecture, *our* examples and *our* program. They say they learned when they attended our classes, or even on occasion worked for us. As a rule, they're just small, local neighborhood groups and they don't hurt us. But we wouldn't mind a credit line.

While I am busy talking to fat people, Al and the rest of the staff (it's grown to more than 400 people in our home territory) take care of the business end of the Weight Watchers organization. There have been close to three million people who have attended classes since 1963, when we started being businesslike and keeping good records. Every week, there are more than 8,500 classes held, with an average of 40–50 members in each. That's over 300,000 people at any one time. In Metropolitan New York alone, we run almost 400 classes a week in approximately 170 different locations.

Isn't it amazing? Isn't it unbelievable that, starting with my little group of six in 1962, all this could happen? I can hardly believe it myself. That's why I hang on to pieces of myself, so I won't forget what went on before all this— the egg candler, my fat dress, the framed red pouch, my first letter from a fan, pictures of me with famous people, pictures of me when I weighed 214 pounds.

Chapter Twelve

IT'S A LONG WAY FROM the basement in my house, where I started. I'm in a world I never dreamed was possible for me—hobnobbing with movie stars and TV performers, running around the country and talking to thousands of Weight Watchers members, appearing on radio and TV, receiving keys to cities and being greeted with brass bands.

I don't lecture to classes anymore. That's become impossible. But I do make public appearances in all the cities and countries where we have locations. I schedule an appearance about twice a month and so I am constantly traveling. We hire a large hall, which will hold maybe 1,500 to 2,500 people, and then invite members and the public to hear me speak at no charge. Anyone may attend if we can fit them in. That's one of our problems, fitting in all the thousands of people who come. In New Jersey recently, 3,500 people crowded into a hall and we had to turn hundreds away. In Louisville, Ky., in Toronto, Canada—everywhere, it's the same thing.

It's thrilling to talk to such huge audiences. When I was in London last year visiting our location there, I gave a lecture to hundreds of people. When I was through, a woman came up to me and said, "I feel like I've met the Queen."

Another woman told me, "Mrs. Nidetch, you were a smashing bomb." At first, I didn't know how she meant that, but then I was told that, to a Briton, a "bomb" is the greatest. And "smashing" is even better!

I was quite nervous about speaking in England, but, you know, I stood up there and I forgot all about talking to English people. I was talking to fat people who sat there with the same look on their faces I'd seen in California and Pennsylvania and Texas. The same look I'd seen in the

Bronx. That same hopeful look. When they stood up and applauded at the end, I fell in love with England and its gracious, charming people.

I kept thinking, there are classes throughout England now and we are now in Scotland. Look where it all started—in my cellar.

I made an appearance in Woolsey Hall at Yale University recently. It was pouring rain outside, a miserable night, but 2,500 people showed up. After my talk, hundreds of people came up to speak to me, as they usually do. One very distinguished, elderly man came up, took my hand and started to say something. Then he began to cry.

I was so surprised that I was speechless for a minute and then I said, "I don't know if you're crying because you've been successful in Weight Watchers or because you're sorry you've spent the evening here." I thought I'd make a joke of it.

He said, "God bless you. My daughter was a hopeless case, but she joined Weight Watchers in Florida. I wish you could see how beautiful she looks today." He kissed me and he walked away.

Last year, I flew to Louisville, Ky., for a public appearance and some television and radio interviews. Just before the plane was to land, the stewardess came over to me and said, "Mrs. Nidetch? The pilot has had a message from Louisville that you are to be met by a large group of people. He asks if you would please disembark last, after everyone else is off."

I said, "May I please have that in writing from the captain? I can't believe it."

In a few minutes, she came back with a note from the captain and I started worrying. As I quickly repaired my make-up, I thought to myself, "How shall I act? Should I be Marilyn Monroe going down the stairs? Or should I be Princess Grace?"

I still hadn't decided by the time the other passengers, including my secretary, had all left the plane. I gathered my belongings, put my handbag over my arm and emerged into the sunshine at the top of the ramp.

There below me were hundreds of people carrying signs which said things like, "God bless Jean Nidetch." "Be lean with Jean." "Help stamp out obesity." "Jean Nidetch, we love you."

The whole group was cheering and behind them was a

brass band. A real band, just for me. It was playing *Hello, Dolly!*

Thrilled to my toes, I walked down the stairs and, as I did, my handbag opened and hung there on my arm, its contents falling out all the way down the ramp. When I got to the bottom, a microphone was thrust under my nose and a man asked, "Mrs. Nidetch, how does it feel to have so many people love you?"

I answered, "You know, when I was getting ready to get off the plane, I thought to myself, 'When I go down there, should I be Marilyn Monroe or Princess Grace?' But look at my handbag! Who am I? I'm Jean Slutsky Nidetch of Brooklyn!"

I am still Jean Slutsky Nidetch of Brooklyn, but my life is so different today from what it was eight years ago that it's hard to believe. I feel it just can't be me. Maybe I'll wake up one morning and find myself fat, ugly and unhappy about finding a dress to fit me. Maybe it's all a dream.

I used to wake up in the morning and feel for my hipbones, because if the bones were there, I wasn't fat. And if I wasn't fat, it wasn't a dream. It was really me, lying there, an imperfect size 12.

But I've enjoyed a slim life for nine years and I can barely remember that fat one. I can look at my own fat pictures now and I sometimes think of the person I see there as "her." I am getting used to being thin.

When I walk into a dress shop now, I go to the size-12 racks without thinking about it. Five years ago, the thought was so thrilling, my heart would palpitate. But now, I'm so accustomed to being thin that I have to force myself to recall how I used to feel. The only time I'm very aware that I was fat is when food is put in front of me and I have to think, "Can I eat that?"

But I don't want to forget that I was fat. If I forget, I may get fat again. If I forget, I won't be able to help other people solve their weight problems because I won't know how they're feeling. So, I put on my fat dress, the size 44, more often than I used to. I put it on and I tell myself, "I used to wear that dress and it was tight on me." I wear that dress and I can remember the despair of those days.

I pray that I'll never forget where I came from. I pray I'll never get to the point where I'll think I've always been thin, successful and at the end of the rainbow. I have to remember the bottom, because I could slide down again so easily. That's why I wanted to write this book, because it's becoming more and more difficult to remember a life before Weight Watchers, before the moment I met that girl in the supermarket in September, 1961.

This book also gives me a chance to communicate with thousands of overweight people who haven't been reached before, people who need encouragement and help. Perhaps, with the information they find here, they can help themselves or come to us.

I want to hold on to the memory of how I felt in the beginning of this adventure. Those were great days when I first started Weight Watchers; it was like walking into the wilderness. I didn't really know what was happening, but I enjoyed every minute of it.

Other people didn't know what to make of us, either. The landlord of our building in Little Neck didn't know at first if he wanted to rent the space to me. He wasn't sure what I was doing up there. So, he'd come up to see what was going on and why all those people kept streaming in and out all day long. I don't blame him. Today, he's very happy to have us as a tenant.

I miss the early days when everything was such a challenge and a struggle. I wanted the landlords to say, "It's a pleasure and a privilege to give you a room where you will do so much good for so many people." But they only asked how much we were willing to pay and how many people would be wearing out their stairs.

I wanted a fat person to say, "I'm going to your class because I am sure I will be successful here." Instead, they used to say, in effect, "Show me. Prove to me that you can help me." Today, there is no more doubt. People join because they *know* it works. And, in a way, I miss the doubting. I enjoyed convincing people of their own power over themselves.

The early success was fun, too, though I found it hard to believe, sometimes. I used to play games with people. I'd walk into a shop to buy gloves and I'd say, "It's such a delight to try on gloves now that I have slim fingers." (I'd always had slim fingers, but I had to open the conversation somehow.) I'd say, "I never used to have slim fingers. I used to weigh 214 pounds."

The salesgirl would look shocked and she'd ask, "How did you lose all that weight?"

And I'd answer, "I joined an organization called Weight Watchers. Have you ever heard of it?"

She'd usually say, "Yes, and I've heard great things about it. It's marvelous."

And I'd feel like I'd had a cool drink on a hot day.

I would go home and tell Marty and he would warn me, "What you're doing is fishing for compliments. One day, you'll meet someone who won't give you the right answer. You better stop doing that."

But I had to do it, just to get the feeling that I was really helping people and was appreciated for it. And to prove to myself that I really was thin.

I'd open up conversations by saying, "I just love trying on clothes now. When I was size 44, it was no fun."

Or I'd say to an overweight waitress, "I'd like half a grapefruit, please. You know, I've joined a weight reduction club. I don't know if you've heard of it. It's called Weight Watchers."

Then I'd sit back and wait for the comments. I'd never tell people who I was. It was more fun if I didn't.

I shouldn't admit it, but I still get a thrill out of the same kind of thing. I was in the Boston airport a few months ago with Marty and a couple of the men from our foods division. The plane was delayed and we decided to have something to eat in the airport restaurant.

The waitress came up to the table and I said, "Do you have fresh fruit salad?"

She said, "Yes, we do."

I insisted, "Are you sure it's fresh and not canned?"

She answered, "I'm sure. It's cantaloupe and honeydew and orange and grapefruit, all fresh."

"Okay," I said, "and I'll have some coffee, no sugar or cream."

When she brought the fruit and coffee, the waitress said, "Are you a member of Weight Watchers?"

I said, "Yes. In fact, I've lost 72 pounds. I used to weigh 214."

By this time, the men in my group were cringing, but I kept a straight face.

The waitress answered, "Oh, how marvelous. I belong, too. I've lost 20 pounds and I've got 25 more to go. I have twin daughters who are 17. One is thin and the other is heavy. The heavy one joined Weight Watchers, too, and she's lost 40 pounds. It's marvelous."

One of the men whispered, "Go on, tell her who you are."

But I didn't. I was glad she hadn't recognized me because then her story wouldn't have been such a compliment. It was like hearing a beautiful compliment about your child from someone who doesn't realize she's talking to his mother. So I sat there and enjoyed the moment.

Of course, I enjoy recognition. I am delighted when someone greets me on the street. I love it when people rush over to me and kiss me because Weight Watchers has changed their lives.

Let me tell you a story. I was invited to speak at a lunch in Asbury Park, N.J. It was the Annual Award Convention for members of Weight Watchers in New Jersey to honor 100-pound losers and give them their Certificates of Accomplishment. There were 120 of them in the area, plus three 200-pound losers.

Marty and I left New York about 8 in the morning in order to be there at 11. The day was glorious, the trip was delightful and I was thrilled to be meeting all those successful New Jersey Weight Watchers members.

As we got out of the car in front of the hotel where the lunch was taking place, we saw many people entering the hotel wearing corsages and boutonnieres. I knew these must be the 100-pound losers who would be honored that day. But no one said hello to me.

I said to Marty, "They don't know me! They've lost weight with us and they don't know me." They had to be Weight Watchers members because there was nothing else going on at that hotel that day. But nobody spoke to me.

By the time I walked into the dining room to be greeted by the New Jersey area directors, I was very depressed. I said to them, "Those people don't know me. Haven't you told them about me? I started this whole thing—and nobody spoke to me!" I was feeling very sorry for myself.

I went into the ladies' room and was standing at the mirror fixing my hair when two girls walked in wearing corsages. Neither one said hello. I couldn't bear it another minute.

I said, "I'm Jean Nidetch."

One of them said, "Of course. We know."

And I said, "Well, for heaven's sake, why didn't you say hello?"

She answered, "I guess we were afraid. We didn't know if you wanted to be bothered with us."

It was a whole new picture. They were in awe of me. I couldn't believe it.

So I said, "Please, let's talk. I want to know, how long did it take you to lose the 100 pounds? How long have you had it off? What size did you wear when you started? Have you had much trouble staying with the program? What size are you today? You look so marvelous and I'm so thrilled for you. But, you know, I feel like my mother would feel if I walked past her on the street without speaking. Do you suppose everybody in this place feels like you do? Is that why nobody has spoken to me?"

She said, "Of course. Everybody knows you, but they're afraid to approach you."

So I walked back into the dining room and said to one of the area directors, "You've got to let me get to that microphone and talk to these people before I burst. I've given them so much of myself and I desperately need to have them know me. Just to *know* me, not to thank me. I can see the thanks in their appearance and their attitude. But they can't *ignore* me. I want them to know what I feel for them, that I'm here and nothing could keep me away on such an occasion. I'm not a television performer. I'm not an author or a movie star. I'm me. I'm Jean-who-was-fat!"

I went to the microphone and told them how glad I was to see them looking so good and how they had nearly destroyed me by not feeling free to come up and say hello.

I decided right then that I must travel even more than I had been. I *must* meet all the members of Weight Watchers wherever they are. I *must* have personal contact with them. I miss it. I don't have the time to run a class myself anymore. I used to know every member, his problems and his hang-ups. I'd meet someone on the street and before I'd remember his name, I'd remember his Frankenstein—I knew whether it was pizza or peanut clusters or Danish pastry.

Today, I have to learn about the classes from what the lecturers tell me. Even if I visit a class, I don't find out what's happening because, when I walk in, everything stops. They want *me* to talk

Other things have changed, too. Naturally, Marty and I and the boys—as well as everyone else connected with

Weight Watchers—have a lot more income than we had when Marty was driving a bus. We can go out now and not have to worry about being able to pay a baby-sitter. We can go to Europe if we like, or on a cruise to the Caribbean. We can take time out for Florida when the winters seem too long. I can buy clothes without first looking at the price tag.

We've moved from our apartment in Deepdale Gardens, the place with the cellar, to a house four blocks away. When we decided to buy a home, I didn't want to leave the neighborhood where I'd lived my fat life. I felt that my life was changing so much in so many other ways, I didn't want to make a drastic break. There is pleasure in taking small steps.

I wanted the boys to remain in the same school district and to have the same friends. I wanted to be able to shop in the same supermarket where I met the girl who told me I looked like I was due. Marty wanted to stay in his same gin rummy game and to feel like the same man. We wanted to tell our friends and neighbors we hadn't changed.

A boy came up to me one Saturday night while we were having dinner with some friends at our country club. (Country club? Do you know, I never knew anybody who belonged to a country club. And now, I belong to one. I had never even heard of country clubs until a few years ago. In my family, rich was if you lived on Long Island. I didn't know about people who went to Europe or sent their kids to camp.) The boy said, "Mrs. Nidetch, I just want to touch you to see if you are real. I lost 40 pounds on the Weight Watchers program. I was ashamed to let anybody see me before because I was so fat, and I had a speech impediment besides. Now, I'm thin and I don't have a speech problem anymore. When I heard you were here, I had to come over and say thank you."

I turned to the people at my table and I said, "If you've ever wondered what Weight Watchers is, this is it. It's a boy whose whole life has changed because of some encouragement we gave him. This is what it's all about."

Certainly, Weight Watchers has become a big business and because of that, my life has changed. But its real meaning is in the people who come to us to help them solve a terrible problem. Its real meaning is changing the lives of unhappy people so that they can feel comfortable in society. Its real meaning is the boy who is no longer

ashamed to be seen, the woman who has come out of
hiding after 12 years, the man who now dares to ask a girl
to go out, a child who is chosen for the baseball team.

I receive hundreds of letters a week from people who say
things like, "Every night in my prayers, I say, 'God bless
Jean Nidetch.' "

Like, "Being fat is like being a zombie. A fat man spends
his life settling—for a job, clothes, perhaps even for a wife.
Thanks to you, I'll never have to settle again."

Like, "If it weren't for you, I would still be sitting behind 422 pounds of wall. Now I'm within striking distance
of a new life. I've thought about suicide more than once.
I had tried every diet, psychiatry, hypnotism. I would have
let a witch doctor do a rain dance on my chest if he would
tell me that weight would come off. The combination of
love, information, companionship and commiseration of
fellow fat persons I found at the lectures did it for me."

And, "I must be only a single unit among the throngs
who wish to say, 'Thank you.' But, 'Thank you,' is not
enough. I say, 'Bless you.' Bless you for creating a way
for fat people to find a new beginning, for opening doors
for me I never knew existed, for letting me enjoy life."

And, "Now that I've broken the sound barrier—gone
below 200 pounds—I must write to you and tell you how
wonderful I feel. Now, I can stay awake after dinner and
have discovered that plays have second and even third acts.
Now, my daughter's French homework has improved because I am around to help her with it. And I've landed a
job I'm certain I could never have landed six months ago
looking the way I did."

And, "It's wonderful. No more turning sideways to get
through a subway turnstile; no more taking up two seats
on the train; or people doing double takes when I walk
by; or high blood pressure; or catcalls from the boys in
the street."

When I read things like this, I know that I wasn't cursed
when I was fat. I was blessed. I must have been blessed.
If I never had been fat, I could never have helped people. I
was blessed to be fat and angry—and *desperate* enough to
do something about it and then to help other people do
something about themselves.

Chapter Thirteen

EVERYBODY WONDERS what goes on at a Weight Watchers meeting. So I'm going to give you an example of a typical class—shortened, of course. After all, most classes last over two hours. But first, let me explain a few things about the program.

The classes have a maximum limit of 100, but the average class runs from 40 to 80 members. That's a lot of people, but I think if you have too few, a new person feels he stands out. It makes him self-conscious. In a larger group, he's one of a crowd of anonymous fat people. And besides, if there are too few people, the newcomer often feels that something must be wrong. It's like sitting in an empty restaurant—how good can the food be if nobody's there? I don't like to sit in a half-empty auditorium. I think, "Why don't more people come to hear this man sing? You know, maybe he's not so great." He may be the best singer in the world, but that's not the feeling I get.

On the other hand, we don't like to have classes of more than about 80 because everyone must have his chance to talk and to get to know everyone else.

Only registered members may attend the meetings; we don't allow visitors. And no one with less than 10 pounds to lose is accepted because it's demoralizing to members who have greater problems. Besides, we don't want people to come just out of curiosity.

No one who joins Weight Watchers signs a contract. It's up to you to decide whether or not you are benefiting from attending the classes. You may come for, say, seven weeks, and then decide to quit. You don't have to pay for an entire "course." And you may rejoin later, if you want to. To join, there is an initial registration fee; then a weekly charge which you pay when you arrive at each meeting.

New members receive a copy of the rules, the food program, a menu plan and suggested menus and recipes. Most people stick with the program. Some don't, of course, and I like to think they'll come back maybe next month, maybe next year, and finish losing weight. It's a matter of the right timing. If a person doesn't stick with it, he's simply not ready. Nobody can make you join and nobody can make you stay—there's no commitment. Sometimes a person will decide to go it alone and, with the encouragement derived from a number of meetings, will accomplish the weight loss on his own. Wonderful. It's too bad more fat people can't do it on their own—but we're there to help those who *can't*.

There are thousands who think of themselves as secret members of Weight Watchers. They attempt to follow the program without ever joining and this is fine with me. We know that members give the printed program to their fat friends; we are aware of that when they come in and say the dog ate it and they need another copy. I would have done the same. And now, with this book, you won't even have to have a friend swipe a copy for you. It's all right here.

But I feel that owning a copy of this material is nothing compared to the support you find at a meeting. If you can learn that cupcakes and spaghetti are fattening and then manage to stay away from them, you don't need us. But the compulsive eater needs something more than a diet. He needs understanding. He needs a belief in himself. He needs encouragement. And he gets it in the classrooms. Here he finds a haven, a place where no one will ridicule him, where other people are going through the very same struggle.

If you join a group and you find no rapport between you and the lecturer, you may always try another group. There's no extra charge; once you've paid your weekly fee, you may go to any class you like. It's like choosing the right doctor. There's no point having a lecturer you can't communicate with. I think that if our schools worked this way, there would be better results. There are certain years your children excel in school and when you go to Open School Week and meet their teachers, you know why. Other years, when they don't do so well and you meet their teachers, you know why, too. It's not that the teachers aren't good, but they and your children just don't blend. The chemistry isn't right.

Usually, once you find the right lecturer and class, nothing will keep you away. When the East Coast was blacked out a couple of years ago, I received a phone call from one of our lecturers in Brooklyn.

He said, "Mrs. Nidetch, I'm here at the Bay Ridge center."

I said, "That's unbelievable. There's a blackout of the entire East Coast. Why did you go out tonight?"

He answered, "I don't know, but I'm here with a flashlight. There are 17 people here with me and they insist on having a class."

"Well," I said, "I'll see that somebody gets candles to you." So I went through the list of our lecturers and found one who lived near the center. I called him up and he walked over with candles and matches. There, in the dark in Bay Ridge in Brooklyn, they had the world's first Weight Watchers meeting by candlelight.

There was one man who used to reach my class just as we were finishing up. He was a bartender who slept all day and worked all night and he couldn't make it to a class. He'd rush in, get weighed, and say, "You don't have to talk to me. I just want to look at all of you and get the feel of this room. It's going to last me for a whole week. Now I'll be all right. See you next week." And he'd rush out.

One traveling salesman used to weigh in at a drugstore wherever he happened to be each week and then call me. Every week. And that did it for him, as long as he knew someone cared.

In most areas, you may choose the class time that suits you best—morning, afternoon or evening. In some centers there are also twilight classes, at 4, mainly for youngsters who want to go right after school and get home before dark. Each class lasts about two hours.

You may choose a co-ed group, an all-male group, or a teen-age group. In the beginning, only women came to the classes. Housewives. Often, it was a little game for them, something to do for the afternoon, a change from the usual routine. Who else would try anything so unknown but a woman with a couple of hours to kill?

Women often start off as skeptics, even today. The first week, sitting in the back row in her dark glasses, she's going to change the rules. When that doesn't work, she often tries cheating, and then insists there's something wrong with the program.

One girl swore to me she'd followed the program to the letter, but it wasn't working for her.

"Are you sure you're eating exactly what you are supposed to?"

"Yes, exactly."

"Well, just to be sure, I'd like to ask you something. What did you do yesterday?"

"I drove up to Connecticut with the children to visit some friends."

"Did you stop for anything to eat on the way up?"

"Just for ice cream cones for the children."

"That's nice. Did you have any yourself?"

"No, I just bought them for the children."

"Did they eat them all up? Did you, by any chance, finish the cones for them?"

The woman blushed. She said, "Well, as a matter of fact, I did. They'd had enough and I couldn't throw the leftovers out the window or I might get a ticket. And I couldn't put them in the ash tray because they'd melt."

That's the way it goes with the women.

But once a *man* decides to join, he is almost always serious and, frankly, less devious than a woman. He'll wait until he's convinced that it can work. When he joins, it's rare that he doesn't succeed. He isn't kidding. He's giving up an evening of poker and he's not there to waste time. He's desperate enough to give it a chance.

We started the men-only classes because we discovered there are men, usually the very obese, who do not want to be in a class with women. Most men aren't interested in dress sizes or swollen ankles or how to prepare a tasty dessert. A man certainly doesn't want to hear about menopause. He wants to sit in a room with other men and talk straight from the shoulder about losing weight.

The men-only classes started about six years ago when a man who had lost 65 pounds with us told me he'd love to be a lecturer. He is a lawyer and a persuasive talker, so we decided to try it. We passed the word around that this class was for men only and on opening night, about 60 men joined. I wasn't at the meeting because, by my own rules, no women were allowed; the weigher and the clerk had to be male, too. But Marty was there and so was Al Lippert. They reported that the average weight of the members was approximately 300 pounds and there were some who weighed over 400.

By the way, I've noticed that when a very large man loses his initial 50 pounds or so, he often transfers to a co-ed group.

I occasionally receive an invitation to attend an all-male class and what always strikes me is that the truckdriver is sitting next to the doctor and the barber is talking to the schoolteacher. Nobody asks a new member what kind of work he does, because it doesn't matter. They're all overweight, that's what matters. They all speak the same language and have the same problems. They're interested in things like, "What's your bad hour?" It's like asking a mother what her baby's crying hour is. Everybody who is a compulsive eater has a bad hour. For most people, it's in the evening after dinner.

Or they talk about how long they've been fat. Or whether their wives cooperate. As the weeks go on, members find out more about each other.

One man will stand up and say, "When I'm driving my cab all day, it's hard to park and go in somewhere for a substantial lunch. I used to grab anything I could get. I'd stop at a diner and order a piece of pie and a glass of milk. But since I've been coming here, I take the time to eat properly."

Another man will say, "I happen to be a doctor and I probably know more about nutrition than anyone in this room. But this is where I learned how to lose weight."

In one men-only class, I was told, a man stood up and said, "Gentlemen, I am a surgeon. I was performing an operation yesterday and the trousers I've been wearing for years in the operating room suddenly fell down! My hands were busy and I couldn't do a thing about it. But I was so proud that I didn't have that big stomach holding my pants up, it didn't matter a bit. I finished the operation in my shorts."

"I remember," said another man, "all the years of getting dressed in the morning and being quite convinced that this was the day I was going to choke to death because the collar of my shirt was getting so tight."

And still another said: "I wonder if any of you know the experience of bending down to pick up something and having the seat of your pants split right in half. It's been used as a joke by comedians but, let me tell you, when you weigh 300 pounds and it happens, it's no joke. The same with having a chair break under you. That happened to me last year and I couldn't get up off the ground without the help of four people."

Men want to lose weight for the same reasons women do. They usually start out by saying, "I don't care about my suit size. I just want to lose weight." But when a man does lose, the first thing he'll tell you is, "I used to wear size 50 and now I'm wearing 40 slim." Vanity is a gift given to men as well as women!

Youngsters started to come to classes, too, and joined the co-ed groups. The women in the class would say things like, "I used to wear a size-40 dress. Now I'm an 18." Well, a teen-age boy couldn't care less. The women would say, "I've discovered a fantastic way to cook No. 3 vegetables. I cut them all up and I add oregano and salt and pepper and I cook them in tomato juice." A teen-ager, boy or girl, certainly won't get choked up about that. He's interested in whether his bowling game will improve, whether he'll be able to ride a bike, whether girls will like him when he's thin.

And he's anxious to know if the other kids will still think he's dumb. It's a terrible thing, but the fat kid is often thought to be stupid.

After a while, we decided that teen-agers should be with teen-agers only. By teen-agers, we mean youngsters 15 and under, and the "under" could be as young as 7. At about 16, a youngster starts thinking more like an adult and then usually prefers to enter an adult class.

The teen-agers have a tremendous compassion for each other. They worry about each other and they give each other strength. Youngsters, as well as their elders, need to tell their secrets.

In a teen-age class, a youngster will stand up and say, "Do you know that I have candy bars in my dresser drawer?"

And the other kids in the room will say, "So, what's so terrible about that? We did that, too."

The first boy would never have admitted this before and he feels very guilty about it. But, now, he's found out he's not unique—it's almost standard to hide candy bars in a drawer if you're fat. Not only that, but you have to plot it out. How are you going to get them there? Where are you going to hide them—under your socks? How will you get rid of the wrappers? You can't leave them in your wastebasket, particularly if your mother has been after you. So you take the wrappers to school and throw them out there. It's one horrible experience after another. Does this sound familiar? It's basically the same with all fat people—children, teen-agers and the older, more mature ones as well.

Teen-agers complain a lot and we give them a place to complain. They don't feel free to complain to adults, so they complain in class, where the lecturer and the other youngsters are empathetic.

Mostly they complain about their parents. I don't think they do it angrily, they just want to explain things to themselves. "Why does my mother say, 'Go to class and lose weight,' and then, when it's my birthday, she says she's making a cake and it won't hurt me to have some?" I've often explained to youngsters that, just as it will take a long time for them to learn how to eat properly, it's going to take their parents a long time to learn that if their son doesn't have a cake for his birthday, he is not deprived.

My own grandparents and my mother used to urge me to lose weight, but my grandmother always brought me chocolate kisses and my mother fed me cake and said, "I don't know why you're fat. I never give you butter or fried food." She meant well, but her rewards were always sweets and starches. She wanted me to be happy.

The teen-agers always want to know, at the beginning, "Why can't I have just one potato chip? Is one potato chip going to hurt me?" Well, it isn't. But we just aren't capable yet of eating one of anything. We're going to eat more, just like that TV commercial says. If just one potato chip had satisfied us before, we wouldn't be fat now. The trick is to avoid the first one.

I always remember the child who came to my son Richard's birthday party. I said to him, "Aren't you going to eat the birthday cake?"

He looked at me and he said, "No, thank you, Mrs. Nidetch. I love it, but I'm allergic to chocolate."

I could see he desperately wanted to dig into that cake, so I said, "Suppose we call your mother and find out if one little piece will hurt you." I weighed 214 myself and I couldn't believe a child could pass up birthday cake.

And he said, "No, don't call her because I won't eat it anyway."

Now, if at 4 you can have that kind of courage, why can't you have it at 14 or 40? Why can't you say, "I'm allergic"? Because you are. From chocolate cake you will break out—not in a rash but in fat. And it's uglier and much harder to get rid of.

We do not permit parents to sit in the classes with their children, although we like them to be in close touch with us by phone. Teen-agers want to talk among themselves and they can't do it honestly with their mothers around.

I'm always being asked by parents what to do about an overweight child. My advice is: Of course, you have to provide him with the proper foods and not offer him the wrong ones, but don't keep after him constantly about his eating. He's too close to you to listen and he'll just tune you out. Or he'll eat more in private, which is surely the worst thing he can do. You never know *why* he must eat—it may be a form of rebellion against you and you'll only make it worse by insisting. I remember that whenever my mother suggested I lose some weight, my thoughts would immediately turn to eating. The best thing is to have a relative or friend provide the encouragement.

Another group that's been starting to come to Weight Watchers recently is the extremely obese. These are the tremendously overweight people, the unhappy ones who don't leave their homes, who can't or won't find jobs, who aren't really living in society. Once they do leave their homes and come to a class, a whole barrier has been broken down. There was a man I remember in Miami Beach who lost 145 pounds in a little over a year. When he weighed 311, he was like a vegetable. He never went out. He never talked. His whole life changed the minute he walked into a class where he found understanding and compassion. He hasn't stopped talking since!

Today, it isn't so hard for very obese people to come to us; now they know there's hope for them. It's still hard to make the decision, but once they walk in, they've found hope because they know it has worked for so many people.

When you walk into a meeting room, you first check in with a clerk at a desk near the door. Here you pay your weekly fee.

Next you go to the weigh-in room where your weight is recorded. Nobody's there but you and the weigher, who tells you right away that she's lost weight and shows you pictures to prove it. Your original starting weight is never

mentioned again until you decide to reveal it yourself—
and you may never want to.

You are given a goal weight when you join—the weight
you should reach at the end of the program. Obviously,
you should keep this goal weight in the back of your head,
but it's not something you should really think about. It's
demoralizing to weigh 280 pounds and be told you should
weigh 145. You just won't believe you'll ever make it. So,
simply take one day at a time. Survive today. Today, don't
eat anything that is forbidden; then, tomorrow, don't eat
anything that is forbidden; then, the next day. You'll find
that if you can survive today, you can manage tomorrow.

Take it 10 pounds at a time. And every time you lose
10 pounds, buy yourself something, take a bubble bath,
indulge yourself. Reward yourself—but *not* with food.

After the weighing, you go into the meeting room where
chairs in rows face the lecturer's table. You sit down with
all the other members who are talking and trading experiences, menus, recipes, jokes and companionship. Looking
around and listening, you feel these are your kind of people
with your kind of problems.

I remember one girl who came to us weighing over 400
pounds. She said to me, "This is the first place I've ever
been where I haven't felt like a freak, a complete misfit.
I sat between two other fat women and I felt right at
home."

The lecturer welcomes the group, introduces herself and
then goes on to talk, just talk. The lecturer is not there to
judge you and your particular shape, but to be a beacon
of light, a buoy, to guide you on your way. She (or he)
never embarrasses or ridicules anyone. She talks about
herself, how she was fat and how she lost her weight. She
shows her own "before" picture. She talks about the problems of being fat and the secrets we all share. She tells
stories about people in her other classes. For the newcomers, she explains the program and the ground rules,
and lets everyone know that they're all in this together.

Then, receiving the weight cards from the weigher, she
calls on everyone in turn, announcing the amount lost (or
gained), and asking each person if he would like to say
anything or ask a question. Most people, I've discovered,
like to get up and talk, but it's a person's privilege to have
a little note attached to his weight card saying, "No discussion." Then, his name is not called at that meeting. But

sometimes he'll get up and talk anyway, like the girl who hadn't said a word in class since she'd joined and then one evening said, "I have to tell you this. I'm married a little less than a year and every night when my husband comes home, he brings me candy. We sit in front of the TV and eat it." She began to cry. "He's still thin but I gained 40 pounds this year and he hardly comes near me anymore. Now I'm fat and miserable."

A little elderly woman, who had been in the group for a few months and rarely spoke, raised her hand. I said, "Do you have any advice for this young bride?"

She said, "Yes. Darling, get rid of him!"

Everybody laughed. It was funny and it took the edge off what was happening. Of course, she didn't really mean it, and then we got serious. The only way I know to cope with this kind of situation is to talk, and I suggested that she do just that. Her husband was bringing her candy because he thought she liked it. I told her my own husband used to bring me those peanut clusters all the time to make me happy. She must explain to her husband very seriously that she needed his help and cooperation. Without it, she'd be lost. She did talk to him and he did help, once he understood.

The new people at a meeting rarely say anything at first, though everyone is free to interrupt the lecturer at any time to ask a question or make a statement. Then, after a few meetings, they begin to ask questions, always the same questions others have asked before, but everyone waits patiently for the lecturer to answer because they can't hear the information often enough. "Will I get flabby if I lose 85 pounds?" "Should I do exercises?" "Why can't we substitute ice cream for all that milk?" "I can't eat liver. May I have something else instead?"

After all the questions and answers and discussion of anything anyone wishes to bring up, the class is over for everyone but the first-time members and anyone else who would like to stay. They are given a detailed explanation of the program.

The 16th week after they've joined, by which time we think they have probably begun to develop proper eating habits, each member who has lost at least 10 pounds receives a small pin. When a member reaches goal, she receives a larger pin (men receive a tie bar) with chips reflecting the total weight loss. I always tell people when they receive the award that if they cheat, the pin will turn green and fall off. Although we never take back the awards even if people regain what they lost, I've received them in the mail from people who wrote: "Please hold this for me. When I lose my weight again, I'll send for it."

The pins and tie bars are so distinctive that people always ask you about them, and so you're constantly reminded of your new way of life.

I know many men who wear their tie bars even when they aren't wearing ties—I guess it's so they won't forget that they are not really cured of being fat.

Chapter Fourteen

AND NOW, here's a partial transcription of an actual class which took place recently:

LECTURER: *I want to welcome you all here tonight. Will all the new members please stay after class so that I can go over the program with you in detail?*

Let me introduce myself. My name is Mildred L. I lost 40 pounds with Weight Watchers. Here's my "fat" picture. That's me in a bathing suit at the beach. I don't know how I could let anyone take my picture when I looked like that.

I've lost 40 pounds and I've kept it off for three years.

For those of you who don't know my story, I'd like to tell you a little about myself, what my problem was and how I came to Weight Watchers. First, I was fat. I was fat my entire life from the time I was born. I had a mother who loved me fat and who loved the rest of her family fat. Her greatest pleasure in life was to feed us. Both my parents thought I was gorgeous, but after a while I began to realize it wasn't so nice to be fat. If I had 100 fingers, I couldn't count the number of times I was called a big fat horse by the kids in the neighborhood.

I thought I was supposed to be heavy, I thought it was hereditary. But I did try to lose weight. I'd go on all those diets you've already tried, but after a while I almost accepted the way I looked.

The other night, I looked at movies taken in 1953. Let me tell you, if you think it's bad to look at a still picture of yourself, it's really horrible to see yourself in motion. I never realized, as bad as I felt about it, that I looked that terrible. My husband always resented it when anyone called me fat, but when he looked at those movies taken in 1953 right after we were married, he said, "Did I say you weren't fat? Call up whoever I said it to. You were fat. You were very fat."

And I got heavier. My mother kept telling me I looked fine and that size 20 was a lovely size. My friends were all thin and I was the mother image to them. I was the one who always held the coats while they tried on dresses. I was the one who minded the baby carriages while they shopped. I would tell them, "I'm not going to look at clothes until I lose weight. I'm on a new diet." It got to be 10 years and I was still waiting to buy clothes.

Finally, I went to a doctor who gave me some mysterious medicine to help me lose weight, and one night soon after I started taking it, I became completely paralyzed. I couldn't move. My husband called the family doctor, who insisted that I go off the medication immediately. Of course, I did, and I decided that I would just stay fat.

But you can't just stay fat. You get fatter. I'm sure all of you are heavier than you ever intended to be. I'm sure you're all disgusted with yourselves. I'm sure you remember always being on a diet.

All fat people say they don't eat much. We think we are different from thin people because thin people can eat anything and we can't. If I asked you all a couple of questions, I'd get the same answers from all of you. Did anybody start a diet on a Friday? Did anybody ever start a diet on a Saturday? Or a Sunday? It's always a Monday, of course.

Now, what happens if you aren't so good Monday morning, if you make one mistake Monday morning? That's right. You've ruined the day, you can't start a diet in the middle of the day, so you eat anything in sight. You'll start again the next morning. If you're not so good on Tuesday, the whole week is shot. You'll start next Monday. If next Monday turns out to be a holiday, well, you'll wait for the Monday after. If you have an argument with your husband, you'll put off the diet for another few days. If it's your father-in-law's birthday, your birthday, your child's birthday, your parents' anniversary, you forget the diet.

For those of you here who joined Weight Watchers tonight, I want you to know the program started the minute you got weighed in. I'm sure that before you came here tonight, you ate up a storm. You ate everything in the house. I know you did it because I did it. The week before I knew I was coming to Weight Watchers, I went wild.

It's been three years now since I joined Weight Watchers.

I have a friend who lives in my apartment building who was a size 16 three years ago. She was going to join with me, but she's still not sure about it. She's still deciding. She's always going to start next Monday. Every week, she tells herself that next Monday she will join, so she eats for the entire week. By now, she's a size 20.

One week soon after I became a member, I lost three-quarters of a pound. When I met this girl, she asked me, "How much did you lose this week?"

I said, "Three-quarters of a pound."

She laughed, "You paid to lose three-quarters of a pound?"

The next week, when I lost a quarter of a pound, I was afraid to bump into her. But I want you to know, nine months later, when I met her with all my quarter pounds and half pounds—40 pounds lighter—she said, "Don't come near me. I can't stand you."

And I was delighted. This was what I'd been dreaming about all my life. I was thin. I'd waited through all those quarter pounds and I was thin.

I'd been dieting for 20 years, but I joined Weight Watchers when I was 36 years old. I sat in the last row in the last seat. I didn't know what I was doing here. I didn't really think that this was the answer, but I just had no other place to go. I couldn't let myself be fat any longer. I'd heard people talking about Weight Watchers, so I thought I'd try it. But I thought to myself, "I'm as smart as anybody else. Why do I need someone to stand up and talk to me?" I listened to the lecturer; I listened to her talk about eating in the middle of the night. She said that if we went to sleep at 2 in the afternoon, we'd all be skinny.

Of course, that was true. Fat people don't eat when anybody watches them. In front of other people, we're great. We're always on diets and we never eat. But we never get any thinner. We eat at night and we don't eat one piece of anything.

We don't intend to eat so much. We only mean to have one taste, one little piece of cake. It looks so good. How is this going to hurt me, one piece of cake? But we never stop with one piece. We never stop until we've eaten the half gallon of ice cream we bought for our child. We had to buy half a gallon because it was a bargain. So we take one spoonful of ice cream and smooth the top out so nobody will notice it. Then we take another spoonful and smooth that out. We keep eating and smoothing and smoothing and eating till the whole container is empty.

We're not like thin people. They don't think like us and they don't eat like us. A friend of mine went to a wedding last week. She's a size 10 and she'll never be anything else. I said to her, "Sally, how was the wedding?"

She said, "It was delightful, but they served dinner very late."

I answered, "So what? What about the hors d'oeuvres?"

"Oh, that!" she said. "I wouldn't waste my time on that garbage."

If I ever thought that hors d'oeuvres were garbage, I'd be thin forever.

Why does anyone come to Weight Watchers? One girl in my Thursday class says she's taking an interior decorating course, but she's decorating her own interior. And that's what we're doing. If we're concerned about what color the rug is in our living room, if we worry about our hair and the color lipstick we wear, we've got to be concerned with what we're putting in our bodies.

There isn't anyone here who has lost weight who could possibly say that it wasn't worth everything he has done without. What are we really giving up when we come here? We're giving up nothing but fat. If our lives have resulted in nothing more than the anticipation of a piece of chocolate cake or a dish of spaghetti, it's pretty sad. It's worth giving up the cake and the spaghetti to be able to live again.

Joan, stand up and tell us a little bit about your experiences. How much have you lost?

JOAN: *Seventy pounds—and it feels wonderful! When you're fat, you don't wear slacks around the house because you look ridiculous. I wore housedresses. I washed and ironed them myself and took great pride in how they looked. One day, I was very busy and I said to my daughter, "Would you please iron my blue dress? I'm in a real hurry."*

She said, "Oh, Momma, your dresses are so big and they take so long to iron."

I couldn't look at my own dresses on an ironing board after that. It seemed to take an hour to iron one of them. Now, it's a pleasure to iron. And I wear slacks, too.

LECTURER: *When people used to describe us, they used to start with our size. It was always, "Oh, you know that girl on the sixth floor. You know, that fat girl, the red-head." Or, "The teacher, the fat one with the pale complexion."*

JOAN: *That's right, and just one other thing. When you're fat and people ask, "How much do you weigh?", you always make the number as small as possible. But, now, I'm not ashamed to say that when I came in here, I was 261 pounds. This is the first time in my life that I ever told anyone how much I really weighed, including my husband.*

LECTURER: *Of course. I always said 150. I really weighed 185.*

Esther, you've been a member for how many months? Five? Esther has been with us for five months and has lost 90 pounds. Tell us how it feels.

ESTHER: *I've never felt better in my life. Just exactly one year ago, I had to break a very important appointment because I couldn't walk. I couldn't walk across the floor. I thought I had broken bones in my feet. The doctor told me it was just my weight.*

I'll never, never gain that weight back again because now I feel that life is so much more important than food. I think I was just eating for something to do, but now there are so many things to do. I bought a dress the other day— I still wear a big size, but I was so pleased to find that the petite department had the same style dress. That never happened to me before. Joan talked about ironing her dresses. Well, besides being so big, mine used to get dirty while I was ironing them because the skirts were so full that they would drag on the floor before I'd get them finished. . . . It's a different life now.

LECTURER: *It is a different life, a completely different life. But remember, we have a long road to go. In order to lose 10, 20, 40, 50, 150 pounds, we have to lose one pound first. You've got to start somewhere. It's the same as getting fat. It didn't happen overnight. You have to stick with the program and lose your weight the right way. How fast you lose it isn't even important. You're learning control and discipline. You'll learn to be selective.*

Bob, how long has it been since you reached your goal weight?

BOB: *Ten months. I originally lost 46 pounds. I gained some of it back and so this week I rejoined.*

LECTURER: *How much did you put back?*

BOB: *Sixteen pounds.*

LECTURER: *Have you been coming here every month since you lost the original weight?*

BOB: *No.*

LECTURER: *That's a mistake. You mustn't think you're ever going to be cured of being fat. Is there anyone here who has never lost weight before? Just one? That's not many out of almost a hundred people. The rest of us have lost weight many times, and every time we swore we were never going to put it on again. But we did. You know, Bob, you have to have gained two pounds before you gained 16. When you gained two pounds, you should have been frightened. You should have come back to the meetings on a regular basis or joined a maintenance class.*

BOB: *I'll tell you one thing, it's very easy to put that weight back on.*

LECTURER: *Of course, it's easy. Very easy. But unless you're frightened, unless you know you have a sickness that you'll never be cured of, unless you're selective about the food you eat and don't go back to your old eating habits, you'll be right back where you started.*

You've got to stick with it. After you've lost your weight, you can eat cake again. But it's got to be one piece of cake. One dish of spaghetti, not the whole pot. And you've got to be guided by your weight gains.

When you've gained two pounds, that's when you should be concerned, because two pounds becomes four, four becomes six, six becomes eight. We're always putting things off in our lives. It's always next month we'll do something, or after the first of the year or before the summer. But that's not the intention here. We must keep the weight off forever, so we can lose it for the last time. Bob, I think you should join a maintenance class after you've lost your weight again.

George, did you want to say something? Stand up and tell everybody how much you've lost.

GEORGE: *This is my 15th week. I graduate next week. I've lost 33¾ pounds. There's a man who works for me who has put on three pounds in the last few months. Now he intends to take it off. As a fat man, I find it rather interesting to hear how he intends to take it off. For the next two or three weeks, he'll give up his afternoon piece of cake. He's done it before and for him it works. All he's doing is cutting out one piece of cake. He's a lucky man, he's a civilian.*

I think there's a lesson to learn there. You have to know exactly what you're eating, to begin with. When you've lost the weight, you have to eat the same amount as you did when you were losing, but add a certain amount to it. If by adding that certain amount you can maintain your weight, then you know you've obviously been successful. But if you don't know how much you're eating to begin with, if you have no control over it, I don't think it's possible to control your weight for any period of time. That's how I understand it.

LECTURER: *You're right. We must never forget that we must always follow the program. Always. If we start cutting out the breakfast and eating cake instead of lunch, it doesn't take very long to forget the entire concept of the Weight Watchers program. You watch yourself. If you're continuing to lose weight and you don't want to, you add a little bit more food. If you're gaining, you take away food. But in most ways, your program stays the same. Our new maintenance classes will help you find the right balance.*

Here's Thelma. She's now employed by Weight Watchers as a clerk. She's one of our prize graduates. Tell the group how it happened, Thelma.

THELMA: *This Sunday will be two years that I'm a member. It's 13 months since I reached my goal. I've lost 109½ pounds and I've maintained my weight for 13 months, isn't that something? It's wonderful to reach a time in life when you feel you were not meant to be wallowing in an ocean of fat. This is the first time in my life that I could go to the closet, choose a dress which I bought last year and be able to wear it. Do you know what it is like to be born at a mature age? I'm starting all over again, and it's a wonderful feeling. It's so sweet, sweeter than any confection you can eat, to be wearing a size 12 after a 48.*

LECTURER: *Isn't that great? Now, having found the answer, don't give it up. Don't let it slip through your fingers. There isn't a piece of candy or a dish of lasagna that's worth it. You must admit that the minute it goes down, you're sorry you ate it. You hate the way you look, so you eat a little more.*

But you're all looking for the answer or you wouldn't be here tonight. Are you willing to give up a caramel? Are you willing to give up a pretzel, a potato chip? Are you willing to throw away your child's leftover food instead of eating it? Are you willing to throw away cold mashed potatoes, pieces of half-eaten bread? If you're willing to do that, you'll make it.

You've got to want to lose weight so badly that you can taste it. That's what you're going to taste, the feeling of being thin. Not the taste of cake. After the first bite, you don't even know what you're eating, anyway. You're just shoveling it in. We're that kind of people.

Now, let's eat everything we're supposed to eat on the program. Let's not love it. We don't have to love it, but we have to eat it because it's going to make us thin. You know something? The thinner you get, the more you like everything, the better everything tastes. Tuna fish tastes better to me now than it did two years ago. It keeps me away from the stuff that's fattening. String beans don't even taste so bad. They're still not great, I'm not mad for them, but I like this white dress I'm wearing. Could I have worn a white dress when I was fat?

Are there any questions?

QUESTION: *How much bouillon are we permitted?*

LECTURER: *As much as you like. It's unlimited.*

QUESTION: *Are we allowed to have dried prunes?*

LECTURER: *No. Dried fruits are forbidden fruits.*

QUESTION: *Can we have the same fish for our five fish meals, or must they be varied?*

LECTURER: *The selection of fish is up to each individual. But it is preferable to eat a variety, basically because this is a long-range program and, if we eat the same thing over and over again, we will probably get bored.*

QUESTION: *How can you get people to stop pushing food at you?*

LECTURER: *You can't. You can only resist. If you resist long enough, they'll stop.*

QUESTION: *How long will it take me to lose my weight?*

LECTURER: *Each person's body works at its own pace. Like snowflakes, no two people are alike, and therefore no two people will lose the identical amount of weight in the same amount of time. Accept the way your body works and be grateful that you can lose weight in any amount while you're eating so well.*

QUESTION: *Do you recommend powdered skim milk?*

LECTURER: *Most container milk still has a percentage of fat. Powdered non-fat skim milk contains none. Also, most people eat in restaurants occasionally and skim milk is not easily obtainable. Nor is it portable. But you can always carry the powdered milk with you.*

QUESTION: *I can't finish all my food at dinner time. What should I do?*

LECTURER: *There are many foods on the program that are not a must. They are merely fillers. If you are consuming these foods—bouillon, gelatine, tomato juice, extra helpings of unlimited vegetables, for example—you can eliminate these items and just eat the basic "must" items. Then you will probably be able to finish your dinner, which you must eat at one sitting. Splitting meals isn't allowed.*

QUESTION: *If you don't feel like eating vegetables as snacks, what else should you eat between meals?*

LECTURER: *You could drink part of your milk in a Weight Watchers shake. You remember, put some milk in a blender, add ice and some flavoring like vanilla extract or instant coffee or strawberries—and you've got a great snack. Or, have you tried the Weight Watchers gelatine recipe? It's wonderful, it really is. It's a great help for those of us who crave something sweet at night. Try grating celery into it. Once it's in gelatine, celery loses its identity completely and it's just crunchy—it could be anything. Make believe it's nuts.*

Now, if there are no more questions, I'll go through the weight cards.

Sue, you gained a quarter of a pound this week. That's not much, but watch it. Sue has lost 200 pounds with us, and this is her first month for keeping her weight loss. Cut down a little, Sue, and you'll have no problem.

Mary, you lost four pounds your first week. That's wonderful. Did you have any difficulty? None? Good.

Remember, everybody, Halloween is next week. If your children come home with candy, get rid of it. Get it out of the house.

Margaret, this week you've had the largest single weight loss you've ever had. How much have you lost altogether now? Fifty-three pounds? Beautiful.

You know, everyone, you never really know when the weight is going to come off in large amounts. Sometimes, you reach a certain point in your weight and you just stay there no matter how careful you are. Sometimes, you may even gain a little. But don't worry about it. Soon, you'll break out of that plateau.

Ann, you've lost a quarter of a pound this week. Well, that's all right, but maybe you can do better. Have you been cheating? A little? Well, you can't do that, you've got to get with it 100 per cent.

Here's what one girl in another class did—she took a full-length photo of Gina Lollobrigida, but pasted a picture of her own face on it. She taped it on her refrigerator so that she would always remember what she was going to look like.

Mary Jane, you've gained a pound. I'll give you a diary. Write down everything you eat. Everything, every bite. I want to know. You may not be cheating in terms of eating the wrong foods, but you may be following the program incorrectly. Let me check it out and we'll find out what it is.

Bernard, your first week with us and you've lost seven pounds. Isn't that great? Are you eating all five fruits every day? That's very important. People tell me they sometimes have trouble getting to eat all the fruits. I remember visiting neighbors one night and the husband said, "You'll have to forgive me if I eat in front of you. It's getting late and I still have two more fruits to go."

Grace, you've gained a little again. What's the matter?

GRACE: *I think I have a mental block. I've been thinking about it all week. I only have 12 pounds to go to my goal weight and I think I don't really want to lose them. I think it's because I will miss coming to the class every week.*

LECTURER: *We'll always be here. You can continue to come back every week or go to a special maintenance class until you can keep your weight loss and then every month for all the bolstering you need. You've lost 33 pounds, don't stop now. As one member said, the time passes anyway, whether you're losing weight or not.*

Good night, everyone—except the new members. Would you please stay a little while longer so that I can go over the program carefully with you?

Chapter Fifteen

MOST OVERWEIGHT PEOPLE, when they try to lose pounds, eat too little. They think they must starve. They think they must suffer a lot. They take a sliver of roast beef and an apple and say, "I'm on a diet." By 9 o'clock in the evening —if they're lucky enough to last that long—they're hungry . . . and now anything goes, right down their throats.

You can never break bad eating habits by being hungry. You must avoid hunger at all costs. On the Weight Watchers program, you can lose weight by eating six (or eight, if you're a man) ounces of roast beef and three or more green vegetables and a cup of bouillon and a tossed salad and two glasses of milk shake and a baked apple— and it's all perfectly "legal"! You walk away from the table filled up and delighted with yourself, and you don't have to worry. You'll lose weight. Besides, you can eat this way the rest of your life. You can't drink oil and evaporated milk or other crazy concoctions the rest of your life. You can't eat only grapefruit and black coffee the rest of your life.

We know that the compulsive eater *must* eat. We realize that food is everything to him. Because we recognize this fact, we can help him lose weight in spite of it. Those on the Weight Watchers program *eat*. We eat a lot, often much more than we ever ate before. We are free to nibble all day long. We may eat compulsively and constantly, just as we always have. But we lose weight. That's because we eat in a disciplined, regimented way, three meals a day, plus snacks. There are over 25 "free" vegetables we can eat, for example, in unlimited quantities. We learn how to re-place the wrong foods (the fattening foods) with the right foods (the non-fattening foods). We may eat all we like, but not what we ate before, not the foods that made us fat.

133

The body needs food for refueling. When you let your car run out of gas and you get stuck on the road, you'll take any gas you can get. But if you put gas in your car when you've still got a few gallons left, you can afford to be selective about the brand you buy or the service station you stop at. The same with food. If you put food into your stomach before you are ravenously hungry, you can be selective. If you wait until you are famished, then anything will do just so long as you're chewing.

We use the positive approach. I often think, "This is the first time in my life when I *must* eat three meals a day in order to lose weight. I *must* eat two pieces of bread a day. I *must* drink milk. I have to eat in order to lose. Isn't that great?"

In order to follow the Weight Watchers program properly, there are certain unbreakable rules you must follow.

• The first rule is that *you may not skip any meals.* That means you must eat breakfast, lunch and dinner. Skipping breakfast has always been the fat person's claim to good dieting. I can never remember eating breakfast unless I was at a hotel and it was served to me. In my own kitchen, breakfast made me sick. But we insist that you eat breakfast, a substantial breakfast. Whether you want to or not is unimportant. There is no rule that says you have to enjoy it. It doesn't have to be the high spot of the day. You just have to do it. Breakfast, this meal fat people never ate, is the most important meal of the day. It's the meal that starts you off and provides ammunition against going off on a binge at 4 in the afternoon.

And you must eat lunch, and then dinner. If you feel hungry at 10 or 11 at night, your hunger can be satisfied with the permitted snacks or one of your fruits or some of the milk you must have. I can't say a green pepper or an asparagus stalk tastes like chocolate layer cake, but either one is quite satisfying and won't make you fat.

Skipping a meal is dangerous for anyone who wants to lose weight. Not physically dangerous, but mentally dangerous, because if you skip dinner at 7, you'll be famished by 11 and you'll eat all the wrong foods. You know how it is. Anything that doesn't move is eligible for your stomach because you're hungry, you're undisciplined and you've been so good. You're entitled.

But, now, you have no excuse because *you do not skip meals*.

• The second rule is that *no substitutions are allowed*. Nothing may be eliminated from the prescribed plan and nothing may be added. Nothing may be changed. We do not allow bargaining. Bargaining is a game people always play with a new diet, but now the program must be followed to the letter. No muffins in place of the bread. No cake instead of the fruit. No ice cream for the milk.

Bargaining has been the downfall of dieters throughout history. If you start by substituting a roll for two slices of bread, you will undoubtedly substitute a sliver of cake for the roll and then a chunk of cake for the sliver.

• Rule number three is *no calorie counting*. It's a trap. If you try to lose weight by calorie counting, you'll discover that you'll select foods by whim, choosing the ones you prefer instead of those that are nutritious. You may lose some weight, but you won't learn how to eat properly or how to maintain your weight loss. If you find, in that little book you have to carry around with you all the time, that a chunk of cake is worth 200 calories and a full lunch is worth 250, you think, "Why can't I have the cake and save the extra 50 calories for later?" But you have to remember that your desire for fattening food is what made you fat in the first place. You have to change that desire or you'll soon be right back where you started.

Besides, if you're like me, you'll get all confused about the number of extra calories you have to play with. You can't live the rest of your life counting calories. You just can't keep it up.

So, we don't count them. We simply follow a program that contains foods we can safely eat the rest of our lives. Obviously, we lose weight because we are consuming fewer calories than before, but we are not tormented by endless decisions and endless counting. We eat what's on the program. Period.

• Rule number four is *no alcohol*. We disapprove of alcohol not only because it's fattening but because it dulls your thinking and makes you forget how to be selective with what you eat. Two or three drinks can make you feel sylphlike. They can make you forget you are fat.

You need a clear mind when you're a compulsive eater. You need to be alert, so alert that that dangerous weapon called your hand doesn't slip too much food into your mouth.

Don't worry about pressure from your friends. Order Vichy on the rocks with a twist of lemon. No one will know the difference. It looks like a martini. Or a Bloodless Mary, which is a Bloody Mary without the vodka. I can get drunk today just by putting on a size 12. That, instead of a 44, can be as intoxicating as two cocktails.

• Rule number five is *no appetite suppressants*. Many people have lost weight that way, but we usually find that they revert to their old eating habits when they go off the pills and gain their weight back—plus some more. Pills are just a temporary crutch and they work for some people but not for the compulsive eater who simply *has* to stuff food into his mouth. And, besides, it has never been our intention to suppress the appetite—we're eating more food now than we did before. In some of my first classes, I used to collect all the members' appetite-killing pills and put them in a big jar on my desk. They were very pretty. One year the women in one class made collages out of them and I have a portrait of myself done entirely in yellow appetite-suppressant pills.

Now to answer some of the questions we hear most frequently.

Why do you recommend weighing only once a week? Because your weight normally fluctuates from day to day and has nothing to do with real gain or loss. I remember when my son David was an infant, one of the very first things I bought was a scale and the very first advice I got from the pediatrician was to throw it away. He said, "Get rid of that scale and stop worrying. Let *me* weigh the baby and be the judge of his condition when you bring him to me."

Most people, when they go on a diet, give up one dessert and jump on the scale. They expect to find that it was worth three pounds. When they're disappointed, they figure, "Why should I give up desserts when I don't lose anyway?" It takes a lot of courage to turn down a piece of strawberry cheesecake, and rejecting it may even make you feel weak and dizzy. But you won't lose 10 pounds because of it, at least not right away.

So, just stick to your once-a-week weigh-in. It's much easier on the nerves. Besides, the ordinary bathroom scale sometimes tends to be erratic. It isn't always accurate. At Weight Watchers, we have professional scales which are accurate—even if you weigh over 300 pounds.

How long will it take me to lose my weight? That's a question we hear all the time and it's impossible to answer. It took me a year to lose 72 pounds. It's taken other people four months, and others, two years. All on the same food. We can't give guarantees. We don't say, "You'll lose X number of pounds if you stay on the program four months."

We just don't know how much you'll lose in how long a period. Our program is not designed, in any case, for very fast weight loss—it's designed to last the rest of your life.

I remember a set of twins who joined. They were employed in similar jobs. They worked together, lived together, ate together. They weighed about the same when they came to us. After four months, one had lost 40 pounds and the other, 20. The only conclusion I could come to is that the body of each twin reacted differently to the foods.

The amount of weight loss and the length of time it takes is also determined by the amount to be lost and by how long the person has carried the excess weight. The person who has 15 pounds to lose will lose less each week in the beginning than the person who has 115 pounds to go. In other words, the very obese individual will lose more quickly than the less obese, at least at first. (It's easier to cure pneumonia than a cold.) And weight which has only recently been put on will be taken off more easily than weight which has been there for a long time.

Will I get flabby if I lose weight? All I can say is I've never seen anyone who ate three substantial meals a day on our program end up ugly. You may be the one exception—I can't give any guarantees. I lost 72 pounds and perhaps I should be flabby, but I'm not. I was so delighted, anyway, to be losing the weight that it never occurred to me that my thighs might be less firm. Naturally, when I weighed 214, my arms and legs were firm and well packed—but with fat. The weight loss is such a joy that, frankly, I have never been concerned about the fact that my thighs are a little less firm than they used to be.

Many people, especially women, assume they will develop wrinkles and sagging. I always say, "What makes you think wrinkles are worse than fat? If you're upset about fat, go ahead and lose the weight. If you look worse when you're thin, it's a simple matter to get fat again."

With our gradual way of losing weight, people don't seem to become saggy. When I starved myself on crash diets, I looked terrible, drawn and miserable, and flabby as well. I also didn't feel well. That was because it was an abnormal way of eating. But when you lose weight slowly, eating the right foods, you give your body more chance to adjust.

When I lose weight, does my stomach shrink? That's like asking if your stomach shrinks once your baby is born. It does get smaller, but it can get big again—all you have to do is get pregnant. If you fill the stomach with enough food, it's going to expand and so will your hips and everything else. But if you keep the food under control, then it's going to stay flat and small.

Should I exercise? If you like to exercise, that's fine. But if your only sport is bridge, that's okay with us, too. Should you exercise while you're on the program? It's entirely up to you. I suggest doing what you've always done. In other words, if you have always exercised, continue to do so. If you never have, don't start now. Concentrate on one thing at a time—your biggest problem right now is choosing the right food. Don't give yourself a reason to get discouraged. Although I believe that exercise is great for muscle toning and general well-being, it won't help you lose weight—the only way to do that is to reeducate your eating habits. Exercise can help you reduce in "spots," but it takes an incredible amount of jumping around to lose just one pound. When you lose your weight, you may then become an exerciser even if you never moved a muscle before. When I was 214 pounds, I didn't look so good in leotards, so you *know* I never exercised. Just the thought of it made me hungry and if I ever did anything energetic, I had a new excuse for eating. Now that I've lost the weight, I'm learning to play tennis. Golf, too.

You should never try to combat two compulsive habits at once, either. If you want to stop smoking, wait until you've learned to eat properly. Make the decision as to which compulsion is more disturbing for you at this time and forget about the other for now.

Chapter Sixteen

HERE IS THE Weight Watchers food plan for weight reduction. Read it carefully because you must follow it to the letter:

INSTRUCTIONS

Weight Watchers strongly advises its members that they consult with their physicians before embarking on this or any other food plan to lose weight, and that, where required by local law, a doctor's certification is necessary.

1. Eat only food listed in quantities specified.

2. UNLIMITED FOODS—Use as desired the following items:

bouillon, approved dietetic carbonated beverages, coffee, herbs, horseradish (red or white), lemon, lime, mustard, pepper, salt, soda water, soy sauce, spices, tea, unflavored gelatine, vinegar (including wine vinegar), water.

3. UNLIMITED VEGETABLES—These vegetables may be eaten raw or cooked, without fat or salad oil dressing, either at meals or between meals. Eat all you want of the following:

asparagus, bean sprouts, beet greens, broccoli, cabbage, cauliflower, celery, Chinese cabbage, cucumber, en-

dive, escarole, fennel, green and red pepper, kale, kohlrabi, lettuce, mushrooms, mustard greens, parsley, pickles (no sugar added), pimientos, radishes, rhubarb, sauerkraut (no sugar added), spinach, summer squash (examples: caserta, chayote, cymling, patty pan, scalloped, straight or crookneck, vegetable marrow, zucchini), string beans (French-style), watercress.

Bonus: 12 ounces tomato juice per day, if desired.

4. LIMITED VEGETABLES—Vary your selection of the following vegetables from day to day (4-ounce serving):

artichokes, bamboo shoots, beets, Brussels sprouts, carrots, eggplant, green beans, okra, onions, oyster plant (also known as salsify), parsnips, peas, pea pods, pumpkin, scallions, winter squash (examples: acorn, banana, butternut, Hubbard, peppercorn), tomato, turnips.

5. FRUITS—Women eat 3 a day, men and youngsters eat 5 a day. One fruit a day should be a vitamin C fruit. Portions:

½ medium-size grapefruit = 1 fruit
½ medium-size cantaloupe = 1 fruit
¼ medium-size fresh pineapple = 1 fruit
2-inch wedge honeydew = 1 fruit
½ cup berries = 1 fruit
Others: 1 whole fruit (medium size) = 1 fruit

You may eat any fruit in season except avocados, bananas, cherries, dried fruits, grapes, papayas, mangos, watermelon.

6. MEATS, FISH AND POULTRY—Broil, pan broil, bake or roast meat, fish or poultry. Do not fry. Remove all visible fat before eating. Do not eat gravies or sauces. Eat at least 5 fish meals weekly. (Everyone is allowed 4 ounces of cooked meat, fish or poultry at lunch. At dinner, women and youngsters are allowed 6 ounces; men, 8 ounces. When buying meats, fish or poultry, allow 2 ounces for shrinkage

plus 2 ounces for medium-sized bone per portion.) The following meats and fish are permitted:

abalone, bass, bluefish, bonito, brains, butterfish;
carp (fresh), chicken (remove skin before eating), clams, cod, crab meat, eels, finnan haddie, flounder, haddock, halibut;
liver, lobster, lungs, mackerel, mussels, oysters, pheasant, pike, rabbit;
salmon (canned), scallops, shad, shad roe, shrimp, sturgeon (fresh), sweetbreads (calf or lamb), swordfish;
trout (brook or lake), tuna fish (fresh or canned), turkey (white meat only; remove skin before eating), veal, weakfish, whitefish (fresh).

Eat any of the following three times a week (do not pan broil):

beef, frankfurters, lamb, salmon (fresh), turkey (dark meat only; remove skin before eating).

7. LIVER—You must eat liver once a week (beef, calf, chicken, lamb or turkey).

8. BREAD—Eat enriched white or 100% whole wheat or cracked wheat packaged bread in the amount indicated. (For men, 2 slices of bread for breakfast and 2 slices for lunch; for women, 1 slice at breakfast, 1 at lunch; for youngsters, 1 slice at breakfast, 2 at lunch, 1 at dinner.)

9. EGGS AND CHEESE—Cook eggs in shell, or poach or scramble (without fat). Eat at least 4 eggs and not more than 7 per week. Eat cheese as indicated. (Breakfast: 1 ounce hard cheese or ¼ cup cottage or pot cheese, or 2 ounces farmer cheese. Lunch: ⅔ cup cottage or pot cheese, or 4 ounces farmer cheese, or 2 ounces hard cheese.)

10. MILK—Instant non-fat dry milk, or buttermilk (made from skim milk), or commercially prepared liquid skim milk that is not a skimmed milk product nor has

milk solids added. Men and women have 16 ounces of
milk daily; youngsters have four 8-ounce glasses daily. If
evaporated skim milk: 8 ounces for men and women; 16
ounces for youngsters.

You may use some of this milk requirement in your
beverage, or you may drink it at mealtime or between
meals.

11. PROHIBITED FOODS:

*alcoholic beverages, avocado, bacon or fatback, beer,
    butter, cake, candy, catsup, cereals, chocolate, coco-
    nut, cookies, crackers, cream cheese, corn, cream
    (sweet or sour);*
*doughnuts, French fries, fried foods, gravy, honey, ice
    cream, ices;*
*jam, jelly, mayonnaise, muffins or biscuits, nuts, oil,
    olives, pancakes, peanut butter, pies, popcorn, pota-
    toes, potato chips, pretzels, pudding;*
*rice, rolls, salad dressings, sardines, smoked fish or meat,
    soda or ginger ale or cola drinks, spaghetti, sugar and
    syrups, waffles.*

WEIGHT WATCHERS DAILY FOOD REQUIREMENTS

BREAKFAST

*4 ounces orange or grapefruit juice or one-half grape-
    fruit or other high vitamin C fruit (to be counted as
    one fruit)*
**1 egg or 1 ounce hard cheese or 2 ounces fish or one
    quarter cup cottage cheese or pot cheese, or 2 ounces
    farmer cheese*
**1 slice of bread (2 slices for men)
    Beverage (if desired)*

LUNCH

*4 ounces fish (canned or fresh) or lean meat or poultry
    or ⅔ cup cottage or pot cheese or 4 ounces farmer
    cheese or 2 ounces hard cheese or 2 eggs*
*Must be eaten at specified meals.

All you want of No. 3 vegetables
*1 slice of bread (2 slices for men and youngsters)
Beverage (if desired)

DINNER

*6 ounces cooked lean meat or fish or poultry (8 ounces for men)
*1 portion of No. 4 vegetable
All you want of No. 3 vegetables
Beverage (if desired)
*1 slice of bread (for youngsters only)

*Must be eaten at specified meals.

Fruits may be eaten anytime during the day.

OPTIONAL

bouillon, 12 ounces tomato juice, No. 3 vegetables

SUGGESTED MENUS

(The meals below are recommended for women. There are slight variances in portion sizes for men and youngsters.)

BREAKFAST

Monday ....*Poached egg on toast, ½ grapefruit, beverage*
Tuesday ....*1 ounce cheese melted on toast, fresh orange juice, beverage*
Wednesday ..*Soft cooked egg, toast, tomato juice, beverage*
Thursday ...*French toast (W.W.Style), ½ grapefruit, beverage*
Friday ......*Cottage cheese on toast, baked apple, beverage*
Saturday ....*2 ounces salmon, toast, ½ grapefruit, beverage*
Sunday .....*Cottage cheese on toast, orange juice, beverage*

LUNCH

Monday ....*Bouillon, 4 ounces shrimp, toast, approved dietetic carbonated beverage*
Tuesday ....*4 ounces white meat turkey, salad, asparagus, toast, coffee*

Wednesday . .*2 poached eggs on toast, salad (no tomato), tea*

Thursday . . .*4 ounces tuna fish, lettuce, French-style string beans, celery, toast, approved dietetic carbonated beverage*

Friday . . . . . .*⅔ cup cottage cheese, fruit in season, toast, coffee*

Saturday . . . .*4 ounces crab meat, roasted peppers, lettuce, toast, tea*

Sunday . . . . .*4 ounces salmon, lettuce and cucumber, lemon, toast, coffee*

EASY LUNCHES TO EAT OUT

- *2 eggs on toast, plus fruit and beverage*
- *Open melted cheese on 1 slice of toast, plus fruit and beverage*
- *Broiled fish, asparagus, fruit, beverage*
- *Tuna or salmon with salad and lemon wedge, 1 slice of bread, beverage*
- *4 ounces sliced turkey or roast beef with 1 slice of bread, fruit, beverage*
- *Cottage cheese and cantaloupe, 1 slice of bread, beverage*

DINNER

Monday . . . .*Sweet and sour veal balls in cabbage, tomato, baked apple, tea*

Tuesday . . . .*Broiled chicken, cauliflower, peas, coffee whip, beverage*

Wednesday . .*Bean sprout soup, London broil, asparagus, Brussels sprouts, fruit, beverage*

Thursday . . .*Liver broiled with onion and mushrooms, carrots, beverage*

Friday . . . . . .*Shrimp, Chinese vegetables, mushrooms, lemon gelatine (made with unflavored gelatine and approved dietetic carbonated beverage), beverage*

Saturday . . . .*Steak, spinach, salad, tomato, ½ grapefruit, beverage*

Sunday . . . . .*Roast beef, mushrooms, broccoli, salad with tomato, baked apple or fresh fruit, beverage*

ADDITIONAL MENUS

- *Veal stew made with celery and mushrooms, tomato, coffee whip
- *Broiled lobster tail, cauliflower, salad, tomato, fruit, beverage
- *Broiled chicken, spinach, squash, baked apple, beverage
- *Shrimp or lobster, broccoli, gelatine (made with unflavored gelatine and approved dietetic carbonated beverage)
- *Liver made with mushrooms, pickled beets, strawberry whip, coffee
- *Leg of veal roast, mushrooms, cabbage, carrots, baked apple, beverage
- *Crab meat, broccoli, salad, tomato, beverage
- *Veal kabobs, mushrooms, green pepper, tomato, fruit, beverage
- *Trout broiled, kale, carrots, green salad, ½ cup stewed fruit, beverage
- *Turkey (white meat), broccoli, squash, cranberry relish (made with artificial sweetener and approved dietetic carbonated beverage)

SOME EXPLANATIONS OF THE PROGRAM

Eat only the foods listed in your Menu Plan, in the quantities specified and at the meals specified. To be sure you have the right amounts, weigh each portion *cooked*.

You will notice that the food requirements for men and youngsters are a little different from those for women. Where women and youngsters are allowed four ounces of meat, fish or poultry at lunch and six ounces of meat, fish or poultry at dinner, men are allowed four ounces at lunch and eight ounces at dinner. Men and youngsters get two more pieces of fruit than women: five a day instead of three. And they have two more slices of bread.

Youngsters are required to drink more milk than adults, four glasses a day, until the lecturer thinks it's advisable for them to switch to the adult program.

The items which are marked with an asterisk (*) must be eaten at the meals specified and may not be saved for another time.

The spices and condiments listed in the No. 2 grouping

may be eaten in any amount you desire (within reason)—as may extracts. Also, though you may eat onions only at dinner, you may use dehydrated onion flakes anytime.

Vegetables may be canned, fresh or frozen. Those in the No. 3 grouping may be eaten at any time, day or night, and in any quantity. The vegetables must never be cooked in butter or any other sauce.

The vegetables in the No. 4 grouping may be eaten only at dinner. You may eat any number of different No. 4 vegetables at a meal, if you like, but the aggregate total must be four ounces. Along with these, you may eat as much of the No. 3 vegetables as you want.

If you wish, you may have a bonus of 12 ounces of tomato juice a day. Although it is not required, tomato juice makes an excellent cooking base.

All fruits are permitted except for grapes, bananas, cherries, watermelon, dried fruits, papayas, avocados and mangos. The fruits must be fresh, or fresh frozen without sugar. You should have at least one citrus fruit a day. Do not eat canned fruit.

You may eat half a medium cantaloupe, but for any other melon, a two-inch wedge constitutes a portion.

A quarter of a medium-sized fresh pineapple, half a medium grapefruit, half a cup of berries—each of these constitutes a portion. Other than these, a whole, medium-sized fruit is a portion.

You may eat your fruits at any time of the day.

You must have at least five fish meals a week, at lunch or at dinner. The fish not permitted are sardines, herring, anchovies and any smoked fish. Canned salmon or tuna fish does not have to be water packed, but do drain off the oil. Do not add fat in cooking fish.

The No. 6 grouping lists the meats and fish you may eat. The last paragraph in that grouping lists those foods you must choose three times a week—no more, no less. These are comparatively high in fat content. You may eat these at noon or at dinner, but most people have them at night because they are usually favorite foods and the portions are larger for the evening meal.

You must eat liver—calf, beef, chicken, lamb or turkey —once a week.

You must eat at least four, but no more than seven, eggs a week, at breakfast or at lunch.

Where the weight of an allowed portion is given, this means *cooked* weight. Meat and fish weigh less cooked than raw, so always buy two or three additional ounces to allow for shrinkage due to cooking. Also, allow two additional ounces for a medium-sized bone. For poultry, allow two ounces for bones and two ounces for shrinkage. Add two ounces to raw fish for cooking loss and two ounces additional for bones. But *always weigh after cooking*.

The bread you eat may be enriched white bread or 100% whole wheat or cracked wheat. Nothing else. You are not permitted to skip bread at breakfast and double up at lunch—or vice versa. Nor may men or women ever eat bread at dinner.

Instant non-fat dry milk, liquid skim milk, buttermilk or evaporated skim milk may be consumed anytime during the day. Any milk used in coffee or tea or in cooking must be accounted for. Remember that evaporated skim milk is concentrated, so instead of having 16 ounces as you do with powdered or liquid skim or buttermilk, you would only have eight ounces of evaporated. Youngsters should have 16 ounces of evaporated or 32 ounces of skim milk made from powdered skim or buttermilk. Do not use "skim milk products" or skim milk with milk solids added.

The cheeses permitted are cottage cheese, pot cheese, ricotta, farmer cheese and any of the hard cheeses that you must cut with a knife. Nothing designated as a "cheese spread" may be eaten. Cheeses may be eaten only at breakfast or lunch.

In the No. 11 group is a list of foods which may *never* be eaten on the Weight Watchers program. These include all starches except bread, as well as alcohol, fried foods, sweets and foods containing a lot of fats and oils.

Chapter Seventeen

THINGS TO REMEMBER:

• *Weigh your food*. Use a small postal scale or a Weight Watchers scale. People often think that weighing is to prevent a tremendous intake of food, but, on the contrary, it's to prevent an insufficient amount. People are amazed to see how much they may "legally" eat. For example, if you are eating small boiled shrimp, a six-ounce portion (a woman's dinner portion) comes to about 18 or 20 shrimp. You probably never ate 18 shrimp at one sitting before in your life, but now you can *and* lose weight. Before this, the average person on a diet would eat three shrimp and then have some potato salad because she was hungry. We want people to eat the shrimp (for dinner, the men get even more—eight ounces) and forget the potato salad. We don't want you to cheat yourself, so use the scale.

Another reason for using the scale is that it teaches control and discipline. We're the kind of people who never sat down to eat. We took a little out of the refrigerator—a little cheese, a little leftover corned beef, a little piece of cake and maybe a little bit of cold potatoes. We never noticed how much we ate. When you must use a scale, you do notice.

Of course, you can't weigh your food in a restaurant, but after a while, your eye and your stomach will be able to tell a six- or eight-ounce portion of meat or fish. And a restaurant will rarely give you more than you are permitted, simply because you are allowed such a large quantity.

In the early days of Weight Watchers, members would usually buy a kitchen scale. Besides being expensive, it was bulky and always had to be on display on a counter. I thought, "We need something small. What better than a postal scale?" The postal scale has a little platform that will hold a piece of foil or a dish. Subtract the weight of the dish and you know the weight of the food. Every postal scale will weigh anything up to 16 ounces.

A woman in Baltimore wrote me this letter recently: "Being a devoted follower of the program, I was preparing breakfast of honeydew melon and cheese on toast one morning. I opened the drawer and took out the tape measure. I measured a two-inch wedge of melon and cut it. Then I took down the scale and weighed one ounce of cheese. Suddenly, I realized there was someone watching me. It was the house painter, who was painting the outside of our apartment house. He was looking at me in amazement through the kitchen window. He knocked on the window and I opened it. He said, 'Lady, pardon me, but what in God's name are you doing?' When I explained that I was a member of Weight Watchers and I was weighing my food, he was *so* relieved. He'd figured I was cracking up."

• *Eat as much as you like of the unlimited foods.* Most people, when they start on the program, are afraid of starving to death, so they gorge themselves on the unlimited foods. I know one girl who ate two heads of cabbage and a bunch of celery in one afternoon. That's fine. Keep right on eating if you have to, as long as you stick to the right foods. When I was first on the program, I used to eat No. 3 vegetables in amazing quantities. I'd go to a restaurant and order spinach and asparagus and string beans and a double tossed salad to go with my meal, in fear of being hungry for something more stimulating. I'd drink the milk shake twice a day. I walked around constantly filled.

In the glove compartment of my car, I'd carry a can of asparagus and a can opener. I was always thinking that if I got stuck in traffic, I wouldn't want to die of starvation. It was almost like the old fat days when I'd go to visit my mother in Brooklyn. I always took along a bag of cookies or a package of pretzels for the same reason. Now it was asparagus—but it didn't make me fat.

There was one mammoth-sized woman who traveled to our classes in Little Neck from New Jersey every week. For a while, she was so addicted to food that she literally could not stop eating; we recommended that she eat the "free" foods, the unlimited ones on the program, and eat them constantly.

She always carried a few cans of mushrooms, along with a can opener, in the glove compartment of her car. On her way to and from the classes, she would pull off to the side of the highway, open a can of mushrooms and eat them. One night while she was eating, a light flashed into the car window and she looked up to see a policeman standing there.

He said, "Is there anything wrong, lady?"

She answered, "No, officer, I am eating my mushrooms." He looked at her strangely, then got on his motorcycle and rode off.

About three months later, she was parked again and, sure enough, a motorcycle policeman rode up and flashed his light in the car. Before she could say a word to him, he said, "Oh, my God, it's the nut with the mushrooms." And he took off.

My favorite snack is a mushroom dish. You take cooked fresh mushrooms, green and red peppers, celery and bean sprouts and season them with salt and pepper, then add half a cup of tomato juice. Simmer for 20 minutes. . . . Try it.

The idea of the Weight Watchers program is that you must never be hungry. You won't get up in the middle of the night to eat if you've had enough food before you go to bed. If you should happen to wake up because of habit, then have the right foods immediately available. If you don't get up, they'll still be sitting there, and if you do, they will be as accessible as the cookies. If you could plot so much to provide yourself with the wrong foods, why can't you now plot with the right foods?

Most women never wash celery until it's time to eat it. Don't keep it wrapped in the paper it comes in and shove it in your vegetable container. Instead, wash it right away, put it in a jar of cold water and have it sit in the refrigerator like a little bouquet. Then it's ready to grab in the middle of the night. It may not be as delicious as a cookie, but certainly it will solve the problem. Until you break the habit of raiding the refrigerator, at least you can raid it for something that won't harm you.

Or prepare yourself a bowl of Lemon Gelatine dessert for just this eventuality. It's sweet, it's delicious and it's "legal." Eat it whenever you crave sweets.

I always suggest that people cut up all the No. 3 vegetables in a big bowl. Then throw in some cut-up fruit (making sure to measure it first). You'd be surprised how pretty it looks—we call it our "popcorn" bowl. Put strawberries or pieces of apple or pears right in with the cut-up celery, green pepper, asparagus or whatever, mix it up, sprinkle sugar substitute over the whole thing—and nibble all night long if you want to. And I used to think the only way I could fall asleep was to have a can of beer and a salami sandwich!

Everybody gets off the eating kick after a while. You keep stuffing yourself until you realize you don't have to, you *can* survive, you *can* feel good, you *can* feel full. Then, vanity sets in. You like what you see in the mirror and you can now cut back on the quantity of food you eat.

• *Eat only what is on your prescribed list.* We don't get much bargaining in our classes anymore because people know we won't allow any deviations from the program unless their doctor prescribes them. What we get now is, "There's a new product out. Is it permitted?"

If our research department hasn't yet examined the food in question, we have to answer, "We're not sure of the ingredients in many new products, so stick to the 'legal' foods until we have a chance to investigate."

We do not allow dietetic food except for the sugar substitutes and the low-calorie beverages. We allow the sugar substitutes simply because there is no other way—except with sugar—to sweeten food. We allow the soda because of a social problem. If you are holding a glass of something at a party, nobody is going to ask you why you are not drinking. Nobody is going to know that what you are holding is low-calorie ginger ale and not champagne.

To my knowledge, dietetic foods were invented for people who have to limit their intake of sugar. So the dietetic foods eliminate sugar, but they often contain other ingredients which are not allowed. For example, there is dietetic apple pie, dietetic whipped cream and then dietetic cherries that you can put on top of the whole thing. All that's missing is sugar, because, as it stands, the concoction contains flour and oil and nuts, and all the other ingredients of a fattening life.

Besides, one thing leads to another. If you eat the dietetic apple pie, what's going to stop you from discovering dietetic puddings? If you use dietetic salad dressing, what will you do if you are in a restaurant and the dietetic dressing is not available? You're going to rationalize and say "What's a little mayonnaise going to do? It can't put too much weight on me." But it's petty larceny, and that's what leads to grand larceny.

For a salad, we recommend that you use wine vinegar or a lemon wedge, both of which are always available in any restaurant or diner. You get used to eating salad that way at home, and when you go out, it's not a big problem.

We also recommend that you drink skim milk. And, for many reasons, we recommend that you drink the powdered skim milk. One, it's easily available. Two, it doesn't spoil. Three, you can always have it with you, in your purse or your pocket. And four, it helps you discipline yourself. If you get used to using container or bottled skim milk at home, on some occasion you'll find yourself at a friend's house or in a restaurant where there is no skim milk available. So, you'll take whole milk, another case of petty larceny. We don't approve of slipping even the tiniest bit from the rules because you'll then find yourself slipping more and more.

Carry a few packets of non-fat dry milk (dry form) with you, and it will always be ready to throw into a cup of coffee, a glass of ice water or a low-calorie soda drink.

Buttermilk is also permitted, but not everybody likes it. Try combining it with tomato juice. It sounds strange, but it's delicious, great for a midday snack. Certainly better for you than a piece of cake and coffee, which is what you used to have.

• *Don't tempt yourself.* I suggest that you don't keep sweets in your house. If you have to keep looking at a chocolate layer cake or peanut clusters, it's like putting an alcoholic in a distillery. Don't surround yourself with food you know will get you in trouble. If you have children, I'm sure they'll understand if you explain why you can't have cookies and candies in the house just now. Besides, they're better off without them, too. And the dentist will probably approve of, and agree with, the elimination of sweets and cookies for them.

Every afternoon when my son David was about a year and a half, I pushed his stroller to a neighborhood candy store and bought him a malted milk. I didn't get one for myself because I was on a "diet." Now no small child can consume two glasses of malted, which is what you got then in Brooklyn. It never occurred to me to leave the second glass on the counter. I drank it, of course. After all, it was mine, I paid for it.

I've developed a great system for overcoming temptation. I suggest it to anyone whose problem is resisting starchy foods. A girl called me up a few years ago and said, "Jean, I have to talk to you. I'm sitting here and I'm holding a doughnut in my hand. It's been 40 minutes now. I've been fighting it, but I'm losing so I decided to call you. Do something, please!"

I said, "While I'm holding on, wrap the doughnut in a piece of aluminum foil and put it in the freezer."

She answered, "Okay," and put down the phone.

When she came back, I went on, "All right, now, let's talk. Tell me about your children. What are they doing in school?" We talked for an hour. Then I said, "Now, go check that doughnut before I hang up." She came back and said, "It's frozen solid."

I said, "Good, you're safe. You'll never be able to bite that doughnut now."

Later, I discovered an even better way to do it. Hold the doughnut or cookies or cake under a faucet and watch it go down the drain. You know, that's an unbelievable experience—you want to dive right in after it. But it works. Before Weight Watchers, in an effort to lose weight, I used to wash tuna fish to remove some of the oil. Then, if I found a loose pretzel in the cupboard, I'd eat it because I'd been so good with the tuna fish. But I should have forgotten about washing the tuna fish and washed the pretzel instead. So remember, if you feel a cookie syndrome coming on, immediately wash the first cookie you pick up.

While you're on the program, never go to a party hungry. Fortify yourself before you go out—to take the edge off your appetite—because, no matter what, you may not eat "illegal" foods. If you're hungry, you'll be tempted to eat too much, perhaps by a hostess who will badger you to try her chocolate mousse. If you're not starving, you can always tell a hostess who follows you around with a mousse, "No, thank you. I think I'm due for a gall bladder attack. I'd better not."

If you feel tempted to indulge yourself with some forbidden food, indulge yourself another way. After I'd lost my 72 pounds and felt like giving myself a treat that wasn't a banana split or a parfait, I bought a little rubber pillow for $2.49. It had suction cups on it and I'd put it against the back of the bathtub, fill the tub with hot water and some bubble bath, and just lie there. It's a great feeling, a feeling of, "This is my hour. This is the hour I'm doing something for me."

I used to sit down in the kitchen after a rough day and make myself a salami, cheese and onion sandwich, and say, "This is my hour." Well, that was great, but I paid dearly for that hour.

That reminds me of a woman in one of our classes. She was the mother of five children and, until she joined Weight Watchers, she used to eat *after* she'd fed the children. Then she sat down exhausted, frazzled, irritated—and cleaned off everybody's plates as well as her own. At the meetings, she was reminded that if she was going to act like a garbage can, she was going to look like a garbage can. It was recommended that she eat first, before the children, so she could resist the temptation to finish up all the leftovers. She went a step further. She put her food on a tray, added a vase with a rose and carried it up to her bedroom. There she sat and dined liked Cleopatra before it was time to feed the kids. It worked.

• *Make your food as attractive as possible.* All the food permitted and required on our program is good, healthy, wholesome food, and it can be presented in interesting and attractive ways. We have developed hundreds of "legal" recipes using these foods (you'll find plenty in my cookbook).

Felice Lippert and our staff work with the recipes that come to us from members of Weight Watchers all over the world. They test and analyze the recipes to see if they are entirely "legal." They also find the answers to other food questions, such as: Are palm leaves permitted? How about turtle meat? Sassafras juice? When our research staff decides a new food is permissible, it is included in our lists.

Today, new recipes are handed out in classes and a bulletin containing them goes out monthly to every franchise. And *Weight Watchers Magazine* prints lots of "legal" recipes in each issue.

There are many ways to make your food more interesting and satisfying. Aside from new dishes, try eating things differently. A good suggestion is to make open sandwiches with your allotted bread. (If you are a man, you're allowed two slices at a time. If you're a woman, slice your one piece through horizontally with a very sharp knife, making two slices out of it.) Top one piece of bread with half your cheese allotment, or a sliced hard-boiled egg, or two ounces of fish, covered with a piece of lettuce. Then, the other slice the same way. It feels like more that way than if you put all the cheese or egg or fish and two pieces of bread together. And, our way, it takes longer to eat!

Or, if you want to get away from eating sandwiches altogether, which is a good idea, put all your food on a plate and eat it with a knife and fork. Then have your bread with your coffee.

Eating a baked apple takes longer than chomping on a raw apple. It not only tastes better (prepared Weight Watchers style, of course), but you put it in a bowl and pour some skim milk over it and eat it with a spoon and it makes you feel as if you're indulging yourself. You'll be satisfied longer.

It's the same feeling I get when I broil half a grapefruit. The time and effort it takes to broil that half a grapefruit and sprinkle some cinnamon and sweetener on it makes me feel I'm doing something nice for myself.

• *Watch how thin people eat.* I know you get the feeling that thin people always seem to be eating waffles and ice cream, but if you watch them closely, you'll see that they have control. One serving of waffles and ice cream will hold them for a week. And besides, they never finish it. They leave most of it on the plate.

Thin people, when they don't want to eat something, are able to turn it down without a big fuss and the hostess hardly notices. Take a lesson and don't make a big deal when you turn down food. Just say, "No, thanks." If the hostess is insistent, let me tell you what I learned when I had just lost all my weight. A civilian and I were sitting together at a luncheon. I was still one of those people who publicly gives away her parfait. I wanted recognition for having lost weight, so I very clearly told the waiter that I did not eat parfait and insisted that he remove it from in front of me. I noticed my friend took her parfait but she never put her spoon to her mouth. She mixed that ice cream up so it looked like she'd eaten some, and then she put the spoon down. It's a marvelous trick and I've used it many times since.

• *Don't worry if you're not eating at home.* Many people believe that if you eat out much of the time, you can't follow the Weight Watchers program. That isn't true. There isn't a restaurant in the world, from the most glamorous French restaurant to the smallest diner, where you can't get something that is permitted. You can always get canned tuna fish. You can always get hard-boiled eggs. You can ask for fish broiled without butter or sauce. You can usually get Swiss cheese or American cheese or cottage cheese. You can get roast beef. You can get hot dogs. Or broiled chicken.

The restaurants are certainly aware of Weight Watchers by now, and if you order a Weight Watchers meal, I've found that the waiter will usually recognize you as a member and will be happy to help you. If not, order your meal: "Fish broiled, no butter, please." Do it very seriously and he'll bring it to you the way you want it.

Even on a plane, you can get what you want. If you call an airline in advance of your flight, you can get broiled meat without the gravy, salad without dressing, vegetables without butter, and fresh fruit for dessert.

It wasn't always this way. I remember going into a cafeteria and ordering an iced coffee. The man at the counter put a blob of whipped cream on top.

I said, "I'm sorry, but I don't want it with whipped cream."

He got very angry and shouted, "You didn't say no whipped cream!"

I thought, "If I tell him I'm on a diet, he'll still be mad." So I said, "You know, I have 'fatonmythigh' and can't take whipped cream. I'll pass out."

He said, "Really? My uncle has the same thing. He can't eat whipped cream either." And he took back the glass and gave me my iced coffee the way I wanted it.

I thought to myself, "This poor man is going to go home to his wife and say, 'I met a woman today who passes out from whipped cream.' "

Usually we get questions from people who must eat out a lot. But sometimes, it's the reverse. Some women say, "If I could only eat in restaurants and not be subject to the temptations in my kitchen, I could follow the program so much more easily." My only answer to that is, don't have the tempting things in your kitchen! Don't surround yourself with cake and cookies and seeded rolls. If your husband likes seeded rolls, just buy one at a time for him, and remember that it's his.

Wherever you are, the best trick I can suggest is: Do not have a loss of memory. I sometimes wonder what happens to our memories when we are raiding the refrigerator. Have we forgotten the experience in the dress shop when the saleslady had nothing to fit us? Do we forget, when we're using both hands to fill up a plate from a buffet table, that we are standing there tightly corseted and unable to take a deep breath? Have we lost the memory of how winded we became just a little while ago when we climbed a flight of stairs?

Maybe it would be a good idea to hang a mirror, a good-sized one, in your kitchen so you can look at yourself whenever you are tempted to break the rules.

I went on a cruise not long ago and was trapped on an ocean liner where I was surrounded by food. I came off that ship after two weeks having gained only a pound and a quarter. You know what kept me from drowning in that food? The thought that I wouldn't have any clothes to wear coming home.

Chapter Eighteen

LOSING WEIGHT is basic training. It's finding out how to eat intelligently—it's learning how to fight the war. The war really begins, though, once you've become thin. Then you go out into the world where nobody knows you really are fat. People always say, "Underneath that fat body is a thin one trying to get out." But it's also true that when the thin one gets out, the fat one is just waiting for its chance to come back. I could get fat again without a bit of trouble. It wouldn't take me much time at all to gain back 72 pounds.

I don't know of anybody who has been fat who ever feels totally safe again. We know we're not cured. We're merely arrested. We know we can surely be fat again. Just give us a couple of weeks of eating the way we used to. We still want chocolate-covered cupcakes and marshmallow cookies. Don't let anybody kid you that you will ever get sick when you look at food. The best you can hope for is that you will get sick when you look at *fat—yours*. But, sick from food? Never.

By the time you've reached your goal weight, though, with our program, you have learned quite thoroughly which foods are dangerous for a thin body. You've learned a completely new way of life. You've learned to like foods that are good for you, believe it or not. I never flipped over liver, but I still eat it once a week and enjoy it. If I find it's Friday and I haven't had liver all week, I decide there's nothing else I'd rather have for dinner.

My heart never throbbed when I thought of milk. But now, if I'm almost asleep at night and I realize I haven't had enough milk that day, I get up and go into the kitchen to get a glass. But that isn't so strange, considering that I used to do the same thing for half a cake.

Since you'll never be thoroughly cured of being potentially fat, something has to control you once you've lost
your weight—because, though you may like liver now,
you're still going to drool over peanut clusters or pizza
slathered with anchovies and sausage.

Tip number one: I find it helps to carry a "fat picture"
with you *at all times*. When you're faced with a splendid
dessert, take out the picture and look at it. If necessary,
paste one on your refrigerator door or on the kitchen wall.
If you look at it often enough, I doubt you'll ever permit
yourself to get back into *that* condition again.

Tip number two: Keep a dress or a suit from your fattest
days and take it out of the mothballs every so often and
try it on. I put on my size 44 every couple of months and
it's enough of a shock to send me back to the green peppers
if I've slipped even a little.

At Weight Watchers, we have tried to solve the most
important problem fat people have, this problem of keeping
the weight off after we've lost it. We have just finished
developing, through years of trial and error, a Maintenance
Plan that will keep us in our new shape. Never again, if
we stick with it, will we have to pack away the thin clothes
and buy new fat ones with the big pleats in the pants or
the doodads at the neckline. Best of all, we can eat real
people food again.

While the weight-losing part of our program is uniform,
the same for everyone, maintenance is custom-made for
each individual. And although there are rules and regulations to keep you on the straight and narrow, choices are
involved—choices that must be made by *you*.

Before this, if people couldn't manage maintenance on
their own, they'd continue to attend our regular classes to
get help from the lecturer and bolstering from other people
in the same situation. Now, we have special maintenance
classes that are especially for those who have lost their
weight and want to keep it off. After all, once you've
reached your goal, you don't need to hear more about
losing.

I've always thought that when you've lost a lot of weight
and are faced with the problem of which foods you may
safely eat, it's somewhat like standing in a redemption
center ready to cash in the supermarket trading stamps
you've taken months and months to accumulate. The
stamps have been painstakingly pasted in books and now

you are standing there and wondering, "What shall I trade them for?"

Well, I frankly doubt that you would take the first thing you saw. I doubt you'd take a lamp because it happened to be on the nearest counter. If the stamps are valuable to you and they've taken a long time to collect, you're going to be rather careful about what you get for them. You may even walk out and not trade them in at all. I can remember going in and thinking there was nothing there I really felt was worth giving up all those stamps for.

I think the same thing happens to the ex-fat man or woman who is faced with all the goodies that used to be so enticing—and so menacing. You say to yourself, "Well, this is cashing-in time. If I take the hors d'oeuvres, I can't have the dessert."

You must make a choice. You can't take everything or you're on the road back to obesity. It's a matter of being aware. I'm aware when I cross the street that I have to look both ways. It's not much of an effort and I do it because I was taught to do it. My life happens to depend on it and it's the same thing with eating.

So, on the Maintenance Plan, you must make decisions. *Which do I want—ice cream after dinner or a cocktail before? . . . Do I prefer a muffin or a piece of cherry pie?* You know you can't have them all and you know you must stop after one portion. After a short time, this compromising becomes such a part of you that you begin to eat like a civilian, the person who always did know when to stop eating.

Up till now, maintenance was your own problem, even though we tried to help. It was a do-it-yourself method of keeping your weight at goal. You added some of the foods you'd been craving, then took them away if you gained weight. It was all trial and error and some people couldn't make it.

Most of us, I've found, developed little tricks. Most of us stuck to the program Monday through Friday and did our splurging on goodies over the weekends. Some people were able to add extras every day; others couldn't. Some people would go on binges (against our advice, to be sure) for a couple of days or weeks, gain weight, then go "legal" again. But whatever the method, I have to admit it was risky because each person had to wrestle with his own conscience.

That's why we've developed the new planned, step-by-step Maintenance Plan—just as easy to follow as the reducing program. We've tested it with groups of people throughout the country and it works. It will help you gradually get back to eating what you once considered "normal" food (I call it *people* food) without getting fat again. I am on it now, and I tell you, it's fantastic! I no longer eat cake with fear and guilt. I eat it and know I'll be fine. I drink cocktails and my conscience doesn't hurt me—nor do I gain weight. It's great because, after all, we all knew how to lose weight long before Weight Watchers. We needed to learn how to *keep* it off. We managed, but now it's going to be so much easier.

This new Maintenance Plan is almost the same as the Weight Watchers program but with new foods to be added at regular intervals. You eat the type of foods you ate to lose weight, with only a few minor changes, and you choose others from a long list of possibilities that range from baked potatoes and rye bread to cocktails and delectable puddings. You also have a greater choice of both meats and vegetables as well as a wider variety of fruits.

At the end of two months, if you haven't gained weight (and you shouldn't if you've been faithful) you'll know how to eat the people food you've been dreaming about. We have always promised to give back the food you've longed for, and you'll have it.

There are no restrictions about the particular meal at which you may eat a particular vegetable. A whole new selection of fruits is allowed, including bananas and watermelon. To compensate for slightly less meat than you had before, new choices may be substituted—like corned beef, roast pork and even smoked salmon.

The process of adding new foods is gradual. You start off the eight-week program with the suggested menu plan, adding to it from a list of specially popular foods—various kinds of breads, rolls, cereals, potatoes, corn, lima beans, rice, spaghetti, for example.

Next come choices like butter, margarine, cream, salad dressings.

To top this off, after six weeks of maintaining your weight, you may start to add, every single day, a simple dessert such as angel food cake or custard or ice cream.

Then, when you've seen that your thin body can handle

these long-forbidden fruits without disastrous results, there are more marvelous things to substitute into your meals. You'll have to believe me, they're worth waiting for.

One thing's certain: You don't ever have to be fat again.

Chapter Nineteen

NOBODY COULD POSSIBLY dream up stories as powerful as the true stories of some of our successful members. One of our 100-pound losers, a young girl, was married at New York's St. Patrick's Cathedral last fall. She had horse-drawn carriages take her guests from the church to the reception because she felt like Cinderella. She *was*. She lost 120 pounds and her whole life had changed.

When a Weight Watchers member has lost 100 pounds, he joins our 100-pound achievers and receives a special Certificate of Accomplishment. What an accomplishment! Can you imagine what it means to lose that much weight, as much as a whole person might weigh? We've had a number of people who have lost *more* than that, some of them over 200 pounds. These are people who have literally emerged from under a mountain and they feel reborn, alive again. Alive, perhaps, for the very first time.

There are, right now, over 5,000 100-pound achievers, and about 25 200-pound achievers to date, ranging from teen-agers to senior citizens. We're proud of these special groups because they've taken such a long journey and achieved so much.

One woman came to us in Little Neck weighing 340 pounds—she was 5 feet tall. Shortly before she joined, she had attempted suicide because she was so unhappy. She was so fat that her husband had left her and their two small children. She turned on the gas in the oven one night, and was not quite unconscious when someone who smelled the gas called the police. When the ambulance arrived, she could vaguely hear the conversation between the two attendants who were trying to lift her off the floor. Listening to them talk about her as if she was some monstrous freak, she truly wished she had died. They couldn't lift her, so they had to revive her right there on the kitchen floor. Soon after she recovered, she joined Weight Watchers and succeeded in losing almost 200 pounds.

Beverly T. joined Weight Watchers about five years ago. She weighed 450 pounds and has, at this writing, lost 180 pounds. She is down to 270, from a size 60 to size 42, and has 120 pounds to go. You've never met a happier person in your life. She's delighted with herself—though she's at a point where many people start. She told me, "When I was born, I weighed almost 11 pounds, and I was always tremendously fat. In grade school, I was the only one who had to wear a girdle. The best day of my life, up until now, was when I got out of high school because then I didn't have to face the other kids anymore.

"My mother took me from doctor to doctor and I went on all kinds of diets. Once I was put on a 500-calories-a-day diet and one afternoon in high school I fainted. Three boys from the football team had to carry me to the nurse's office. I was so humiliated that I transferred to another school the next day."

Beverly's parents were both heavy, but her sister was thin enough to be a model. "She never understood what was the matter with me. She wouldn't be seen walking down the street with me, I was so grotesque." But she did lend a boyfriend to take Beverly to the senior prom, looking, she says, like two Sophie Tuckers.

When Beverly got married, she had starved herself down to her lowest weight ever—208—but soon started right back up again until she finally went over 400. With no children to take care of, she decided she had to get out of the house and find a job. For a while, she did temporary office work. "In one place," she says, "the whole office staff stood up and stared at me when I walked in. I said, 'I must be in the wrong place,' and left. I went home and cried into a coffee cake."

Then, five years ago, she took an office job working nights after everyone else had left the building. She felt she had to do something, but she didn't want to be around people who would be horrified by her size.

"I never had any friends at all. Never. When I was a child, my only friend was my dog. After I got married, we didn't have any social life either because it was too embarrassing to be around other people. Somebody was always saying, 'Sit on this chair, not that one.'

"I used to drive around the block—I had to have a special oval steering wheel because I couldn't fit behind a round one—past a restaurant, waiting until it was empty. Then I'd go in and eat. Nobody, except the waiters, ever saw me eat. I'd have my husband buy $15 worth of cake and bread every weekend—and it would be gone by Wednesday. Then he'd have to bring me more on Wednesday night. He did it, not because he wanted to—he has always weighed about 142—but because it was easier. There would be no fights that way. Unhappy people have big mouths, you know."

If she dropped something on the floor, it would have to stay there until her husband came home and picked it up for her. Once *she* fell and had to lie there until he arrived.

"It was one awful thing after another," she says. "The last time I got on a bus, the driver asked me for two fares because I took up two seats."

When Weight Watchers came to her city, Beverly called up the center and was told, after she'd explained her plight, "You can't afford not to come." She went and lost 17½ pounds the first week. She also cleared her pantry shelves of five big grocery bags full of "illegal" foods. She lost 80 pounds in 16 weeks and is going strong.

"It's a different me," she says. "I've never been as happy as I am right now. I used to go shopping, park the car right outside the store, go in for one item and come back dripping wet and exhausted. Yesterday, I shopped for hours and felt great.

"I'm going to get a job working days very soon. I'd like to be a receptionist so I can meet people. I'm buying beautiful clothes, and not from a catalog, either. I bought eight things last week and, do you know, not one of them was black! I even bought a shocking-pink sweater. Just think what I'll be able to wear when I lose the rest of my weight!"

Beverly is still a compulsive eater, but she's learned to eat the right things. Like many of us, she keeps No. 3 vegetables in the glove compartment of her car in case of emergency. "That's instead of eating three dozen doughnuts," she says. "Last week, I met a girl I hadn't seen since I was married, when I was down to 208. She said to me, 'You've put on weight.' I got away from her as fast as I could and rushed to my car. I sat there eating French-style green beans until I felt better. Doughnuts are tastier, but when I'm stuffing myself, I don't know what I'm eating anyway. When I go to work at night, I take celery that's cut up into bite-size pieces, and I nibble all night. When I get home at 5 A.M., I have green beans, coffee and a glass of skim milk.

"And I'm getting vain. I always looked neat, but that was all. Now, I'm particular about myself. I worry about my eyebrows, for instance. Who cared before? I'm a walking miracle. It's fabulous what's happened to me."

Two years ago, I received a letter from a man, Henry H., after he'd lost 107 pounds. He's now a weigher for an all-male class. He wrote:

"Weight Watchers took a fat, old, miserable man of 23, and produced a human being. Most of my life I considered myself a freak. I was overweight from the time I was 5 years old. I weighed 120 in the third grade and over 200 when I graduated from elementary school. By the eighth grade, I was so large that at our school's annual dance festival not a single girl wanted to dance with me. As it turned out, I had to dance with another boy who was an extra in his class and didn't have a girl partner. To top it off, I had to dance the girl's part.

"My weight went up and up and up, until about two years ago I reached my high point of 296. I received many nicknames during my fat years, not the least of which was 'Hippopotamus.' I was teased, made fun of and rejected.

"Sure, I tried to do something about the way I looked. I took pills, shots, went on low carbohydrate diets, high fat diets, starvation diets. In fact, I even tried Weight Watchers before, but I wasn't really mentally prepared to lose weight.

"Last August, at close to 279 pounds, I joined Weight Watchers for the third time. The day I joined, I had just finished work and had gone to meet my mother to go shopping. When I met her, my mother took one look at me and started crying. I asked her what was wrong and she said, 'You look like an old, sloppy, ugly man.' As I sat in the store eating dinner, I thought over what she had said. And I thought about the time a year before, when I went up to Canada to visit an aunt I hadn't seen in almost three years. Her first words to me when I arrived at her door were, 'Shouldn't your mother be ashamed to send you here looking like that?'

"After we finished shopping, I went to Weight Watchers. Three weeks ago I received my 100-pound award and to date have lost 107 pounds. To me, the pin represents more than just the loss of 100 pounds. It also means that I have received two very precious commodities—life and a future. Being fat is like being a zombie. You appear alive, but inside you're cold and dead. You sit and watch as life passes you by, but you can never participate in it, either because you are too ashamed or other people won't let you. All a fat man has to look forward to is a life without joy, without promise, without meaning. He spends his life settling for things. Thank God, I'll never have to settle again."

Laurice H., who once weighed 249 and has lost over 100 pounds, said, "It took a fire to start me losing. One night, our house went up in flames. We lost everything, but our neighbors helped us out. They brought a mountain of clothing to us—everybody found something to wear except me. Nobody could provide a size 46. Then and there, I made up my mind to lose weight."

"I knew I was going to die if I didn't lose weight somehow," says Joyce S., a 37-year-old housewife who was the first 100-pound loser in her area in western Michigan. "I was always a big girl, but after I was married and had two children, my weight went up over 200. Finally, it reached 266. About four years ago, I had rheumatic fever. When that subsided, I developed arthritis, which settled in my hips, and my blood pressure went up to the stroke area. The doctor kept telling me I had to lose weight, but somehow I just couldn't.

"Then I had to have major surgery and I was put in a room in the hospital with an old lady who'd had a heart attack and a stroke. She could only move one arm. All I could think of was, 'This is going to be me.' I was 34 and I had a family and this was going to be me. Who was going to take care of my kids after I was gone?"

Joyce remembers swimming in her neighbor's pool one afternoon. It was a very hot day and she and her husband were the only guests, so she put on her size-46 bathing suit and went in. It was a raised pool with a deck all around it and no steps into the water. The two husbands left after a while, then the two wives decided to get out. Her neighbor jumped right out, but Joyce couldn't. "I jumped and pulled, but I couldn't get out. It was so humiliating. I could only think of having to call the two husbands to haul me out. Finally, after bursting all the buttons on my suit, I crawled out."

The last straw came when her son, then 8, came to her

one day and said, "Jimmy says, if you get any fatter, you're going to bust just like a frankfurter."

Joyce joined Weight Watchers. "The night I went to my first meeting, it was the darkest, loneliest night of my life. I wanted to go home and hide. I felt like the fat lady in the circus and I thought there couldn't be others as fat as I was. But there were."

She lost over 100 pounds in eight months and 20 more in another four. Now, Joyce is a lecturer. She says, "I feel I have an obligation to help other people in the same boat. I wouldn't have been alive today if I hadn't come."

Ann W., who has lost 200 pounds with Weight Watchers and still has quite a way to go, told me, "I have a real emotional hang-up with food. The minute I get nervous, I develop an intense desire to eat. Now, I eat asparagus and celery till it's coming out of my ears. Or I cook up a box of broccoli or cauliflower. It used to be bread and cake."

Ann weighed 411½ pounds when she came to us in New Jersey. She had extremely high blood pressure and was beginning to have a sugar problem. Three years before, she had spent two weeks in a hospital on a starvation diet, lost weight, but gained it right back. Like the rest of us, she'd tried diets and pills and everything else, but nothing worked for long.

"I was orphaned at 10," she says. "I was sent to a boarding school for two years and then went to live with an aunt. My aunt decided I was too fat and she locked the pantry so I couldn't eat during the day when she wasn't home. To get even, I went out and bought as much as I could. Food became very important to me. I was 6 feet tall when I was 14, but I weighed over 200.

"When I got married, I was thinner. But as the children came along, I started gaining more and more. We lived with my mother-in-law and we didn't get along. But she was a good cook, so when I got upset, I'd just eat more. Soon, I was over 300.

"After five years, my mother-in-law died and I thought, maybe I can lose now, I won't be so irritable. But it wasn't true. I didn't lose."

Ann's blood pressure finally got so bad and she felt so tired all the time—the minute she sat down after the slightest exertion, she'd fall asleep—that she decided to try Weight Watchers. She didn't think it was possible to stop eating, but other people were having success . . . and besides, there was no other way left.

"The first six weeks, I was miserable. I've heard people say they never had so much to eat as on the program, but I felt starved. I was determined to stick with it for at least 16 weeks, however. By the end of that time, I found I was no longer always desperately hungry. Now, I manage. I still eat all the time—I eat so much celery, you wouldn't believe it. And I'm losing steadily. I can't wait to get to goal so I can splurge a little.

"I still need the encouragement I get at the meetings," Ann goes on, "and probably will for a long time. I need a regular routine where I'm checked and given encouragement. We have a small group and everyone is friendly. They're all always anxious to hear how everyone else is doing. My daughter's joined too and she's lost 30 pounds already. And my son is thinking of it. It's easier when you're in it together."

Margie G. says she's lost a whole person—95 pounds. A friend got into her "fat dress" with her and they were able to button it up with no difficulty at all. "I can cross my legs now. And I take my raincoat off. I always wore it wherever I went. I'm a human being."

When Margie went to camp as a child, she had to sit on the side in a robe during the water shows because she wouldn't put on a bathing suit. "I never did much of anything—just stayed home and ate. I own 14 watches because my husband never knew what to give me. Certainly, food and clothes were out."

The first night Weight Watchers opened in her city, she went, lining up with over 200 other fat people who came to join. She swears she's never cheated on her food since, though "nobody eats as much as I do. At the beginning, I used to eat six or eight cans of green beans a day, then start in on six heads of cauliflower. The grocery man didn't know what to think. But that's all right. I lost weight."

Two weeks after a flight home from Florida, Everett S. joined Weight Watchers. Jammed into a seat next to his overweight wife, 320-pound Everett was unable to fasten his seat belt because it wouldn't go around him, even let out all the way. The plane taxied down the runway to get in line for takeoff.

The stewardess walked down the aisle checking seat

belts. After she discovered his predicament, she walked up to the pilot's compartment and the plane soon pulled out of line, turned around and returned to the terminal. "Here," says Everett, "a skinny guy boarded the plane with an extension for my seat belt. I was so humiliated that I knew I had to do something."

Everett S. was always fat. He weighed over 200 pounds at 13. "I used to have to buy my clothes in the men's departments, and then nothing fit me right. I had a lot of friends as a kid and I thought I was pretty happy. But when I look back, I realize that I never did anything physical nor did I ever go where it was crowded. I was always so uncomfortable in big groups of people. Certainly, I never danced a step in my life.

"When it came to a career, I unconsciously chose one where I'd be working on my own and not have to worry about other people looking at me. I became a research scientist. I was a quiet fellow, never much of a talker. My wife, who was quite fat too, was also quiet."

After that embarrassing air flight, he joined Weight Watchers, and in 10½ months he lost 130 pounds. He's down to 190, which is right for a man just over 6 feet tall. His wife lost 65 pounds.

"I got so enthused over the whole thing," he says, "that I offered to lecture to classes myself. Now, I teach one all-male class a week and sometimes substitute in others.

"I'm a terrible show-off, too. I wear clothes that will make people know I'm there, like a red, raw silk dinner jacket. And we've both learned to dance. We love it."

"I stood in the revolving door of the subway station and the tears rolled down my cheeks," says Pauline J. "I was stuck and I couldn't move backward or forward. I weighed 240 pounds, I was carrying a few packages, and there I was, wedged in like a sardine."

In a few minutes, a man came into the subway station, saw her situation and gave the revolving door a mighty push—and Pauline was free.

"I muttered, 'Thank you,' without looking at him, and scurried into the train that was pulling into the station. At my stop, the first thing I did was stop at a newsstand and buy a candy bar because I felt so terrible about what had happened."

Pauline started getting fat at the age of 7 after she'd

had her tonsils removed. She was a fat child, teen-ager and adult. She never really looked in a mirror, she told me, except to be sure her hair was neat—a quick glimpse that never went below her chin. She wore the most inconspicuous clothes she could find, and only learned about make-up last year. That's because she tried not to think about her appearance, not to admit to being a girl who could be attractive.

"Every day is painful when you're fat. At my fattest, if something fell on the floor in the morning, it waited there until the kids came home from school in the afternoon. My clothes were always too big or too small. I had a wardrobe of dresses, ranging from size 16 to size 24½, one or two in each size. That was because my weight went up and down constantly and nothing fit me two weeks in a row. I was always on a diet.

"I had six miscarriages and each time the doctor said maybe it was because of my weight. So, I'd go on a diet. Once I lost 60 pounds in six months under the supervision of the doctor. At the end of the six months, he said I knew enough to stay on the diet on my own; there was no sense spending my money to come to him every week. I promptly went to a dress shop and bought a size-14 dress, which was the size that fit me then. The next week, my husband and I went on vacation and when we came home three weeks later, I had gained 30 pounds back. In two months, I was up 75 pounds."

Pauline's husband was fat, too. The last time he allowed her to look at the scale when he was on it, he weighed over 260 pounds. That's a lot of pounds when you're 5 feet 8½ inches tall. The two of them would go on diets together, Pauline starting and her husband following a couple of weeks later when he saw that it worked. But the weight always came back.

After two children and a move to Chicago, Pauline was pursued by a new neighbor who wanted to get acquainted. Because the neighbor was tiny and thin, Pauline wasn't interested. Finally, the neighbor managed to get her to come to her house for a cup of coffee. The next day, Pauline invited her back, serving coffee with sugar and cream, and cookies. While the neighbor drank her coffee black, Pauline ate the cookies.

After a while, she said, "I guess that's why you are thin and I am fat."

The girl said, "I'm not thin, I'm fat." Then she told Pauline how she used to eat and how much she used to weigh before she'd joined Weight Watchers in New York, where she had been living. She even ran to her house and brought back some pictures of herself.

"The difference was fantastic," Pauline says. "I'd heard of Weight Watchers before and I'd even seen the program, but I'd never tried it. At that time, Weight Watchers hadn't opened in Chicago yet, but my new friend acted as my lecturer, giving me information, advice and pep talks. It worked. Was I excited! But then my friend went on a long vacation. I was worried about how I'd get along without her—and I didn't. After I realized that I had consumed three boxes of cookies I'd bought ostensibly for the children, I read an ad in the newspaper saying that Weight Watchers was coming to town. I called up immediately. Where? When? I'm coming."

That was the beginning. Pauline lost 102 pounds between July and February, and has maintained her loss for a year and a half. Her husband joined a few weeks after she did and shed 103 pounds. Now Pauline wears a size 10 and even an occasional 8.

"It's been literally a lifesaver for my husband," she says. "His family has a history of heart disease, and the doctor told him if he didn't lose weight he was going to have a heart attack for sure. Now, he's in fine shape. We both are."

Those are just some of the stories.

Reprise

"LISTEN," JEAN NIDETCH said to me one afternoon, "you've got to see this to believe it. I don't mean just in New York, but in Louisville and Minneapolis, in Houston and Detroit and Buffalo and Columbus. If you're going to be the editor of *Weight Watchers Magazine,* I think you should see, firsthand, what Weight Watchers means to people."

I smiled and nodded; smiled because the enormous enthusiasm of this fascinating woman is something to behold and nodded because, let's face it, she was right. I should see it firsthand.

So, a number of us went on trips with her. We traveled to Louisville and Detroit and East St. Louis and West Boondocks—and some small towns, too. We saw thousands of delighted people who came to airports and high school auditoriums and department store community centers and churches and temples to see her and to hear her; to get the word; to be assured that they, too, could rejoin the human race, get back into life, get with it, get thin. They cheered after every sentence and applauded every thought. They laughed when she kidded them because they were fat or had been fat just like she had been fat. They cried when she reminded them that their husbands or wives or children were ashamed to be seen with them when they were ugly and obese, or that they belonged to a cult of stay-homers because they were too fat to get behind a steering wheel or walk up a flight of stairs, or because they simply didn't want to be seen.

They delighted in her energy and burst excitedly with the feeling of confidence she imparted. They had pickets at the airport in Minneapolis; not anti-war pickets but pro-Weight Watchers pickets who waved signs and chanted,

"We want Jean!" On a whirlwind visit to Los Angeles, she did 14 radio and television appearances in two days and found time to sit for newspaper interviews as well and for a dozen chats with people who "just had" to talk to her.

I sat next to her on a flight between Houston and Dallas. She dropped her head on her shoulder and fell fast asleep for 10 minutes. She'd slept two hours the night before. When she awoke, she was ready to go. The pilot came back to say hello and to tell her that his sister went to Weight Watchers. Two fellow passengers heard that she was aboard and drifted by to show their Weight Watchers pins, ask for autographs, exhibit their newly earned thinness.

Once in Dallas, it was more crowds, more interviews, more speeches, more handshaking, much hugging and kissing with people who tearfully declared that they owed their new lives to her teachings. I felt caught up in the emotion of these trips. I sat back, made a few notes and tried to scoff at it, figuring that maybe these were shallow people who needed help. But then, suddenly, I realized that all of us need help from somewhere, somehow, from someone— and that fat people, fat people everywhere, had now found someone they could turn to for their own particular needs.

There were others who thought to scoff, and did. A disc jockey in Florida called her a fraud.

"Why," she asked, "why am I a fraud?"

"Because you scare people into losing weight. You're not a doctor. What right do you have to tell people they ought to lose weight?"

She smiled and looked at him. "I have all the right in the world," she said softly. "I have superb credentials. I was fat. I lived a life of people ridiculing me, of not being able to fit into normal clothes, of not being able to throw a ball to my sons, of feeling ill when I looked at a refrigerator or a smorgasbord table or a candy counter because I knew that, if turned loose, I could eat everything in sight with no compunctions. I have the right to tell other fat people not only that they should lose weight, but that they must lose weight, because *I* was fat and *I* lost weight and *I* saw the difference. I'm not a politician or a preacher or an evangelist. I'm somebody fat that people can relate to. I'm them, 72 pounds later."

"Well," growled the disc jockey, who must have weighed 135 with his overcoat on, "I can't see why people need this kind of help."

But I have seen and, very probably, you have, too. I have seen thousands of people who have been helped by Jean Nidetch and Weight Watchers. For every doubter, I have seen 1,000 believers and another 1,000 admirers. You know what it all boils down to? It's this—we need each other. We have a desperate need for man to help man. There are many kinds of brotherhood. Fat people, sitting in a meeting hall in downtown Duluth and convincing each other that they can do it—that they can achieve what once seemed like an impossible dream—is brotherhood, too. Just ask somebody who used to be fat. And if you really want to know what Jean Nidetch is like, ask someone who has worked with her, who has traveled with her, who has seen her both charged with the electricity of a personal appearance and relaxed in the comfortable atmosphere of her own home with her husband and kids and a black rascal of a poodle named Brandy who likes scrambled eggs, soft slippers and lady poodles, not necessarily in that order.

Have her pull out her 50 some scrapbooks and note the delight she takes in your looking through them. Not just scrapbooks filled with press clippings or photographs with celebrities, but pictures taken back in the '30's and '40's and '50's, birthday cards sent to her children when they were 2, then 3, then 9. Know anybody who's got a program from a Texas League baseball game between the Oklahoma City Indians and the San Antonio Missions in 1948? How about 20-year-old tickets to an ice show in Tulsa or wedding announcements plus all the gift cards from her wedding? Jean Nidetch has hers. She's also got the first corsage her husband ever sent her. It's moldy. Not much left of it, but there it is, neatly pressed between the pages of a scrapbook.

You've got to be a helluva sentimental person to stash away all that memorabilia. You've got to be a helluva person to open your doors to fat women like yourself who want someplace to talk and to meet.

We sat in her den, leafing through scrapbooks, making some notes, looking at pictures, when the phone rang. It was a person-to-person call from a woman in Jacksonville, Fla.

"Look," the caller began, "I've got a complaint. I had to talk to you personally. I went on your program and lost weight. Now, I've gained some back."

The blond hair tossed and the eyes fired. "You," she

said to the voice, "aren't telling me the whole story. How many chocolate bars have you hidden around the house?! How many cakes have you sneaked through the back door? How many big, thick sandwiches have you eaten on the sly?"

I flipped the scrapbook back to the picture of a fat blonde sitting placidly on a Brooklyn beach. "Tell her again," I said to Jean. "Tell her again."

MATTY SIMMONS